Augmented Hypnosis
Multisensorial, multichannel hypnotic techniques.

I0540778

By
Gary Edward Gedall
01/08/2019

Published by:

From Words to Worlds
Lausanne, Switzerland

www.fromwordstoworlds.com

Cover by: Gary Edward Gedall
Cover image, "**No man's land**", oil on canvas by Daniel Will
www.danielwill.ch

ISBN: 2-940535-65-1

ISBN 13: 978-2-940535-65-1

About the Author

Gary Edward Gedall is a state registered psychologist, psychotherapist, trained in Ericksonian hypnosis and EMDR.

He has ordinary and master's degrees in Psychology from the Universities of Geneva and Lausanne and an Honours Degree in Management Sciences from Aston University in the UK.

He has lived as an associate member of the Findhorn Spiritual Community, has been a regular visitor to the Osho meditation centre in Puna, India. And as part of his continuing quest into alternative beliefs and healing practices, he completed the three-year practical training, given by the Foundation for Shamanic Studies in 2012.

He has now, (2014 – 2016), completed a DAS, (Diploma of Advanced Studies), as a therapist using horses.

His hobbies are; writing, western riding and spoiling his children.

He is currently living and working in Lausanne, Switzerland.

By the same Author

Adventures with the Master

Emotional Rescue

The Island of Serenity, Pt 1 Destruction
(Series – published or in preproduction)

Non Fiction - **(published or in preproduction)**

REMEMBER
Stories and poems for self-help and self-development based on techniques of Ericksonian and auto-hypnosis

The Zen approach to Low Impact Training and Sports

The Zen approach to Modern Living
Vol 1 Fundamentals, Family & Friends
Vol 2. Work, Rest & Play
Vol 3 Life Cycle

Picturing the Mind:
Vol 1   Basic Principals
Vol 2   Fields within Fields
Vol 3   Pathology, classical, traditional and alternative healing methods

Disclaimer:

The characters and events related in my books are a synthesis of all that I have seen and done, the people that I have met and their stories. Hence, there are events and people that have echoes with real people and real events, however no character is taken purely from any one person and is in no way intended to depict any person, living or dead.

Contents

Part 1 Hypnosis in General

1. Hypnosis – What is it?

1.1 Introduction to this section

I would imagine that most of the people that have thought to read this book are already; versed in, trained in, and, likely, already practicing the art and science of hypnosis.

However, for those that are not already schooled in this work, here is a micro introduction to some of the basics …

Please note, those that have read, through to the end, of my book on Ericksonian hypnosis, 'Remember', will find most of this chapter in the theoretical section of that work.

1.2 What exactly is hypnosis?

Dr. Gérard Salem (Salem, 2006)[1]
emphasizes that the term hypnosis refers to
three types of phenomena: the hypnotic state
or the trance, the technique used by the
hypnotist, (one might note that leading
someone into or inducing a trance state is
generally referred to as an 'induction'), and
the type of interaction between the hypnotist
and his subject.

1.3 The trance

The trance is considered as a 'modified state
of consciousness', which links the
characteristics of a waking state (as
confirmed by an EEG) with a specific type
of experience of muscle-release/relaxation
and dream-type productions.

---

[1] Salem,Gérard. *Soigner par l'hypnose.*
Éditions Masson 2789 Issy les Moulineaux
cedex 9, 2006.

It is the experience of being here and being there at the same time, (dissociation).

It is a totally natural state which we experience, in principal, about once every ninety minutes; this is a moment of distraction, a pause in our mental processing, when we lose track for a few seconds.

It's as if the mind stops 'to take a breath'. It is also a state that we enter while doing a boring or repetitive task; ironing, washing up, driving, even listening to someone droning on and on and on; many schoolteachers are excellent hypnotists.

What is so fascinating about this state is that we can be totally involved with an experience, with all our senses and yet at the same time be fully aware of our surroundings and be able to react instantaneously. Just think of the situation of driving in a car and daydreaming when someone cuts in unexpectedly; the reaction is pretty much immediate.

Another way to form an image of the trance is to liken it to the feelings just between sleeping and wakefulness; early in the morning when, for instance, one knows that the alarm has rung, that it is time to get up, but one allows oneself just another five minutes to finish that nice, warm dream.

1.4 The suggestion

The suggestion is a key communicational tool in hypnosis, which allows the hypnotherapist to gently lead the subject where he judges it necessary for the subject to go.

1.5 The induction

The induction of the trance is accomplished through two methods:

The first is the use of a constant, monotonous sensorial stimulus (for instance a mark on the wall, the contact of the subject's hand on the material of his clothes or the 'classic' follow-my-watch.

Although not currently used anymore this is very similar to the follow-my-finger technique used in EMDR, see below), on which one asks the subject to focus his attention.

(Yes, strictly speaking, as many of the techniques of induction use an external element, these could also be considered to be forms of augmented hypnosis – see below).

Although, for myself, if I am not using the 'follow-my-finger technique', (even though I very rarely use EMDR, I find this a very quick and effective induction system).

I then tend also to suggest that the patient focuses on their breathing, and this easily leads them in.

This concentration on a specific stimulus reduces, little by little, the awareness of the existence of other stimuli, and the monotonous nature of this particular stimulus provokes a phenomenon of sensorial adaptation which leads the subject to become less and less conscious of it.

Hence, through this process, the attention of the subject turns from the external world to focus more and more towards his inner experiences.

The second method is the use of the voice, and a particular type of communication.

The speed and the timbre of the voice, which, little by little, deepens and slows down, is a very simple and basic part of taking the patient into the other, inner space.

One of the principal tools for the induction and the deepening of the trance is that of the 'body-subject language'.

This is based on a type of verbal formulation within which one refers directly to a specific part of the subject as if it was an independent entity in itself.

One might say, for example, 'maybe your eyes feel that they wish to close' or 'notice how your breathing has become slower and deeper.'

I also often make reference to the subject's body, emotions and mind as if they were independent but linked bodies/entities.

Eeach having their own memories, needs, defences, logic and resources, which, although quite weird as an idea, in practice, proves to have a reality!

The resulting effect is, as noted above, 'dissociation,' (being conscious of the outside reality, all the while experiencing a personal, other reality).

This is an essential characteristic of the hypnotic state.

It also allows the therapist, through a psychological form of 'divide and conquer', to access a specific facet of the patient's psyche, separated from the mass, which might have a different experience of the past, and a different manner of functioning.

2. The History of Hypnosis

2.1 Sources and references for this chapter

The some elements of this chapter are taken from three excellent and very complete works; A Review of the History of Hypnosis Through the Late 19th Century[2], Psychotherapy and Psychosomatics, Development of Psychotherapy[3] and a rich entry in Wikipedia, under the title History of Hypnosis.[4]

To not to overcomplicate the referencing of each citation, especially as one often finds the same sources referred to in several of the works listed above,

[2] D. Corydon Hammond, The American journal of clinical hypnosis · October 2013
DOI: 10.1080/00029157.2013.826172 · Source: PubMed Retrieved 19.05.2019
https://www.researchgate.net/profile/D_Hammond/publication/261101191_A_Review_of_the_History_of_Hypnosis_Through_the_Late_19th_Century/links/552ab1600cf2e089a3aa0ee6/A-Review-of-the-History-of-Hypnosis-Through-the-Late-19th-Century.pdf?origin=publication_detail
[3] Psychotherapy and Psychosomatics, Psychother Psychosom 201 0;79(suppl 1):1–90 DOI: 10.1159/000288804 Published online: May 26, 2010
www.karger.com/pps Retrieved 26.06.2010
[4] Wikipedia, History of Hypnosis
https://en.wikipedia.org/w/index.php?title=History_of_hypnosis&oldid=725837331. Retrieved 01.04.2016

where I have used any one of these three
works, I have chosen to simplify the process
and give only references on the original
sources.

However, I have also used other primary
sources, although I have chosen to not
differentiate between the two, again as
means of simplifying the presentation.

2.2 The Earliest References to Hypnosis

The history of hypnosis more than likely
goes back to the very beginning of time.

In many traditional cultures, there are
practices that create trance states or ASC's,
(Altered States of Consciousness). Fasting,
dancing, rhythmic clapping, drum beating
and the use of hypnotic plants.

Shamanic rituals incite these ASC's, with
certain very clear intentions, hence, for me,
come under the general term of hypnosis.

Timothy Thomason reflects that, "Shamanic and Native American healers have utilized methods to produce altered states of consciousness in themselves and their patients for thousands of years

…. A reasonable conclusion is that since ancient times Native American healers have developed reliable methods to, in effect, hypnotize their patients so they are more susceptible to suggestions that will help them feel better.

This puts Native American healing for psychological disorders on a continuum with modern psychotherapy."[5]

However, according to Will Durant, hypnotism as a tool for health seems to have originated with the Hindus of ancient India.

---

[5] The Role of Altered States of Consciousness in Native American Healing by Timothy C. Thomason, Northern Arizona University, Flagstaff, Arizona http://www.cuyamungueinstitute.com/articles-and-news/the-role-of-altered-states-of-consciousness-in-native-american-healing/ Retrieved 25 06 2019

11

As a form of healing often took their sick to the temples to be cured by hypnotic suggestion or **"temple sleep."**[6]

A practice of staying at night at a temple for meditational self-observance and communication with the gods, was known as **Nidra** in India.[7]

Sleep temples (also known as **Dream temples** or Egyptian sleep temples) are regarded by some as an early instance of hypnosis over 4000 years ago.[8]

In the ancient world, many cultures built elaborate temple complexes dedicated to their healer gods - **Imhotep** in Egypt and **Asklepios** in Greece for example.[9]

---

[6] Will Durant 1997, The Story of Civilisation, Volume 1: Our Oriental Heritage
[7] Shifu Nagaboshi Tomio (1994), The Bodhisattva Warriors: The Origin, Inner Philosophy, History and Symbolism of the Buddhist Martial Art Within India and China, p.398
[8] Cuyamungue, Hypnosis in Ancient Civilizations by David Reeves http://www.cuyamungueinstitute.com/articles-and-news/hypnosis-in-ancient-civilizations/ retrieved 18.07.2019
[9] Ancient Origins, A Dream Cure? The Effective Healing Power of Dream Incubation in Ancient Greece https://www.ancient-origins.net/history-ancient-

12

The ancient Hebrews used meditation with chanting, breathing exercises and fixation on the Hebrew letters of the alphabet that spelled their name for God, to induce an ecstasy state called **Kavanah**.

(These ritualistic practices are very similar to Auto-hypnosis). In the Talmud, Kavanah implies relaxation, concentration, correct attention (motivation)[10]

"Also, in India, yogis and rishis utilized self-hypnosis during meditation to still their minds.

In India, the word hypnosis is referred to as **sammohan**. Sammohan has been practiced in India since the Vedic times, 1500-500 B.C.

---

traditions/dream-cure-effective-healing-power-dream-incubation-ancient-greece-009287 retrieved 18.07.2019
[10] See 9

And also, in 2,000 B.C. **Wond Tai**, also known as the father of Chinese Medicine, wrote about a technique involving chanting and "the passing of hands" over the body".[11]

2.3 The Early Innovators

One of the first important actors in the history of hypnosis was, **Avicenna (Ibn Sina**) (980–1037), a Persian psychologist and physician.

[He] was the earliest to make a distinction between sleep and hypnosis.[12]

---

[11] InfoRefuge. The Early History of Hypnotism. https://inforefuge.com/the-early-history-of-hypnotism retrieved 26.07.2019

[12] Haque, Amber (2004), "Psychology from Islamic Perspective: Contributions of Early Muslim Scholars and Challenges to Contemporary Muslim Psychologists", Journal of Religion and Health 43 (4): 357–377 [365], doi:10.1007/s10943-004-4302-z

Paracelsus (**Theophrastus Phillipus Aureolus Bombastus** 1493–1541), a brilliant Swiss medical researcher, was the first physician to use magnets in his work.

"He wrote at a time when alchemists were beginning extensive studies with metals and he sought to propagate a theory metallic magic to supplement or supplant the older magic which concentrated on empirical herbal lore and angelic or spiritual manifestations.

In addition to his own work on the newly discovered property of magnetism, he served as an influence for Franz Anton Mesmer's dissertation for the doctor of medicine degree."[13]

This was the beginning of a period when the use of magnets became more and more a standard healing treatment.

---

[13] David A. Leeming (Editor), Kathryn Madden (Editor), Stanton Marlan (Editor) Encyclopedia of Psychology and Religion Springer; 2010 edition (October 26, 2009)

2.4 Magnets and Mesmer

Around 1771, a Viennese Jesuit named **Maximilian Hell** (1720–1792) was using magnets… "Among his adventures were experiments in magnetism applied to medicine. …

He met with considerable success in relieving … pain. His magnetic medicine attracted the attention of a young man named Franz Mesmer, recently graduated from the Jesuit University of Dillingen in Bavaria."[14]

Franz Anton Mesmer was born on May 23, 1734, although trained as a catholic priest, he quickly decided to change his orientation and studied to be doctor.

---

[14] Maximilian Hell, S.J. (1720 - 1792) and his Mesmerizing adventures.
http://www.faculty.fairfield.edu/jmac/sj/scientists/hell.htm retrieved 26.07.2019

He believed that there existed a magnetic fluid that existed in all things, including the human body, which he termed "**animal magnetism**".

Hence the use of magnets and iron filings became part of his healing system.

However, he focused his work on patients suffering from psycho-somatic illnesses. His techniques and confident suggestions that the patients would be healed proved to be particularly successful. [15]

2.5 Towards the Modern Practice of Hypnosis

Abbe Faria (1755 – 1819), was possibly the first practitioner to use many of the techniques that we still use today.

---

[15] "Franz Mesmer." Famous Scientists. famousscientists.org. 4 Jun 20 www.famousscientists.org/franz-mesmer/ retrieved 26.07.2019.

Furthermore, his rational was also very much in keeping with modern thought, and totally in contradiction with the magnetists of his era.

He replaced the elaborate rituals of the magnetic movement with simpler suggestive methods, by requesting the subject to close his eyes and focus his attention on sleep. After a short period, he would instruct the subject with one word: "**Sleep**." [16]

2.6 Use of Hypnosis as an Anaesthetic

In the early 1800's, several doctors, **Récamier, Esdaile and Elliotson** reported to have operated on patients using 'mesmeric sleep or coma, as they termed it[17]

---

[16] THE ABBE FARIA: A NEGLECTED FIGURE IN THE HISTORY OF HYPNOSIS, Campbell Perry Concordia University, Canada Hypnosis at its Bicentennial: Selected Papers pp 37-45 November 1, 1978
by F. H. Frankel (Editor) Springer
http://link.springer.com/chapter/10.1007%2F978-1-4613-2859-9_3 retrieved 30 07 2016
[17] William Lockhart, Hypnosis, CreateSpace 2015

Also, during the American Civil War (1861–5) Hypnosis was used by field doctors in the American Civil War and was one of the first extensive medical application of hypnosis.[18]

And in France: "In the year 1847 two surgeons in Poictiers, **Drs. Ribaut** and **Kiaros**, employed by hypnotism with great success in order to make an operation painless."[19]

2.7 Hypnosis becomes a medical technique

"**James Braid** (1795 – March 25, 1860) was a Scottish neurosurgeon who coined the term and invented the procedure known as hypnotism.

---

[18] B. Reid, David . Hypnosis for Behavioral Health: A Guide to Expanding Your Professional Practice. Springer Publishing Company 2012.

[19] Dessoir, M. (1887). Hypnotism in France. Science, 9(226), 541-545. Retrieved from http://www.jstor.org/stable/1762145 26.07.2019

19

He rejected the belief that cures such as those achieved by Franz Mesmer were due to animal magnetism.

He recognized the veracity of the phenomena but believed them to be caused by suggestion.

He developed the technique of relaxation and eye-fixation, known as "**Braidism**," which results in the hypnotic trancelike state.

Braid's work led to the development of hypnosis as a medical technique."[20]

He ascribed the "**mesmeric trance**" to a physiological process resulting from prolonged attention to a bright moving object or similar object of fixation.

He postulated that "protracted ocular fixation" fatigued certain parts of the brain and caused a trance—a "**nervous sleep**" or "**neuro-hypnosis**."

---

[20] New World Encyclopedia. James Braid (physician) https://www.newworldencyclopedia.org/entry/James_Braid_(physician) retrieved 26.07.2019

Braid is credited with writing the first ever book on hypnotism, *"Neurypnology"* (1843).

Braid [also] drew analogies between his own practice of hypnotism and various forms of Hindu yoga meditation and other ancient spiritual practices.

After Braid's death in 1860, interest in hypnotism temporarily waned, and gradually shifted from Britain to France, where research began to grow, reaching its peak around the 1880s with the work of Hippolyte Bernheim and Jean-Martin Charcot

2.8 Europe takes the baton

The neurologist **Jean-Martin Charcot** (1825–1893) endorsed hypnotism for the treatment of hysteria. **La méthode numérique** ("The numerical method") led to a number of systematic experimental examinations of hypnosis in France, Germany, and Switzerland.

The process of post-hypnotic suggestion was first described in this period.

Extraordinary improvements in sensory acuity and memory were reported under hypnosis.

Charcot's pupil, **Pierre Janet**, (1859 – 1947) described the theory of dissociation, the splitting of mental aspects under hypnosis (or hysteria) so skills and memory could be made inaccessible or recovered.

Ambroise-Auguste Liébeault (1864 – 1904), the founder of the **Nancy School**, first wrote of the necessity for cooperation between the hypnotizer and the participant, for rapport.

Along with Bernheim, [**Hippolyte Bernheim** (1840-1919)] he emphasized the importance of suggestibility.[21]

---

[21] See 20

Johannes Heinrich Schultz (1884 – 1970), adapted the theories of Abbe Faria and **Emile Coué de la Châtaigneraie** (1857 – 1926).

Hidentifying certain parallels to techniques in yoga and meditation. He called his system of self-hypnosis **Autogenic training**.[22]

Sigmund Freud (6 May 1856 – 23 September 1939), a student of Charcot, developed abreaction therapy using hypnosis with **Josef Breuer** (1842 –1925).

He also saw it as evidence of the existence of the unconscious. Freud is said to have made use of hypnosis for about 10 years, 1886 to 1896, but he then gave it up for a number of reasons.

---

[22] GoodTherapy Johannes Schultz
https://www.goodtherapy.org/famous-psychologists/johannes-schultz.html

These being; he feared patients would lose contact with the present situation, or become addicted to hypnosis "as though it were a narcotic".

Also he was "anxious not to be restricted to treating hysteriform conditions", and became frustrated because he could not hypnotize all patients nor put them into as deep a trance as he would have liked.

And finally, (and possibly most importantly), one of his patients, "threw her arms around his neck one day on coming out of hypnosis".[23]

---

[23] Rachel Bachner-Melman & Pesach Lichtenberg, Freud's Relevance to Hypnosis: A Reevaluation, American Journal of Clinical Hypnosis 44:1, July 2001

2.9 The American Approach

William James (1842–1910) the pioneering American psychologist discussed hypnosis in some detail in his *"Principles of Psychology".* James recognized the complexity of hypnosis as an interpersonal process. In the end, James' views suggest how a rapprochement between the cognitive and social approaches to hypnosis might be achieved.[24]

In a totally different field, that of 'hypno-obstetrics' **Fernand Lamaze**, (1891–1957) a French obstetrician having visited Russia, brought back to France and then to the UK and finally to the USA, "childbirth without pain through the psychological method,".[25]

---

[24] William James and Hypnosis: A Centennial Reflection John F. Kihlstrom, Kevin M. McConkey First Published May 1, 1990 Meeting Report https://doi.org/10.1111/j.1467-9280.1990.tb00192.x retrieved 26.07.2019
[25] Psychology Wiki History of hypnosis https://psychology.wikia.org/wiki/History_of_hypnosis/ retrieved 26.07.2019

2.10 Russia, Platonov and Psychoprophylaxis

In Russia, a **hypno-suggestive** method was promoted by the psychiatrist Platonov, [**Ivan Yakovlevich Platonov**, (1852-1920)], director of the School of Psychotherapy in Kharkov.

He was interested in the problems of pain and saw the pains of childbirth as a useful area of study. The early procedures, known as hypno-suggestive, caught on strongly after 1936.

By that year, Platonov could report 588 cases treated by him and his associates with about 60 percent success.

A new method, **psychoprophylaxis**, grew out of the favorable experience with the hypnosuggestive method.

It was originated by **Velvovski** and was officially sanctioned by the Ministry of Health of the Soviet Union in 1951, in a publication called ***"Temporary Directions on the Practice of the Psycho- prophylaxis of the Pains of Childbirth".***

Lamaze, as stated above, then popularised this approach in Europe and the U.S.A.[26]

2.11 Hypnosis and Trauma

The use of hypnosis in the treatment of neuroses flourished in World War I, World War II and the Korean War. Hypnosis techniques were merged with psychiatry and was especially useful in the treatment of "shell shock", what is known today as Post Traumatic Stress Disorder.

---

[26] Ernest R. Hilgard, Josephine R. Hilgard, et al. Hypnosis In The Relief Of Pain. Brunner/Mazel Publishers; 1st edition 1994

Two major pioneers in the treatment of traumatised soldiers were **William McDougall** (1871–1944) and **William Halse Rivers** (1864 – 1922).[27]

2.12 Modern Day Hypnosis

The modern study of hypnotism is usually considered to have begun in the 1920s with **Clark Leonard Hull** (1884–1952) at Yale University.

An experimental psychologist, his work *"Hypnosis and Suggestibility"* (1933) was a rigorous study of the phenomenon, using statistical and experimental analysis.[28]

---

[27] Judith Pintar & Steven Jay Lynn, Hypnosis: A Brief History 30 March 2009 John Wiley & Sons

[28] Human Trinity Hypnotherapy Tribute to Clark L. Hull (1952) https://www.paulguydurbin.com/clark-hull.html retrieved 26.07.2019

In the 1940s, **Andrew Salter** (1914–1996) introduced to American therapy the Pavlovian method of contradicting, opposing, and attacking beliefs, and impressed by Clark Hull's little known work in hypnosis and conditioning,

Salter published a seminal paper on autohypnosis in 1941 and a book on the topic in 1944, reporting successful applications to some of the problems (e.g., insomnia, smoking, overeating) he was treating in his newly established practice.

In the conditioned reflex, he has found what he saw as the essence of hypnosis.

He thus gave a rebirth to hypnotism by combining it with classical conditioning.

Using his clinical experiences in a heuristic fashion, Salter went on to publish two other books that form the basis of behavior therapy today,

Conditioned Reflex Therapy (1949) and
The Case Against Psychoanalysis (1952).[29]

Milton H. Erickson (1901-1980).

There are many books written on Milton Erickson and his unique approach to therapy, here are the main elements:

Flexibility. Erickson was supremely flexible, adapting his approach to each individual client.

The second element is working with symptoms to bring about a change. Erickson saw problems as a process, an unhelpful way of going about things that the cient had developed, and symptoms were part of that.

---

[29] Gerald Davison. APS – Association for Psychological Science. Andrew Salter (1914-1996) Founding Behavior Therapist
https://www.psychologicalscience.org/observer/andrew-salter-1914-1996-founding-behavior-therapist Retrieved 26.07.2019

By changing the symptom it's possible to change the entire pattern of the problem.

To engage the unconscious mind by any means available, that the individual's unconscious contained all of the resources necessary to bring about a cure for that individual in the present moment.

Erickson knew that the language of the unconscious is imagination and metaphor, and therapeutic stories, anecdotes, jokes, puns and riddles are a crucial element of his work.

Erickson developed "indirect" or **"conversational" hypnosis.** He also believed in allowing the client maximum freedom to interpret what is being said in their own way, going to great lengths to see the world from the client's point of view.[30]

[30] History of Hypnosis
http://www.historyofhypnosis.org/milton-erickson/ retrieved 07 08 2016

Part 2 Augmented Hypnosis

3. Augmented Hypnosis - The General Concept

As with much in life, it is useful to begin with a clear definition of what we are talking about.

I define Augmented Hypnosis as: *"A form of hypnosis or trance state, induced and, or reinforced by any external aid or device, other than the voice of the hypnotist."*

Is this new?

Not at all.

In fact, what I describe is certainly the most ancient and basic form of trance induction and reinforcement.

So why bother to give it a fancy name and write a book about it?

As a practicing hypnotherapist working both with individuals and running groups, I have, without realising it, been using augmented hypnosis for a long time.

Recently, I have been reflecting on the idea to create an internet-based course, on the broad subject of hypnosis.

I then began to list all the types of hypnosis that I am trained in, and that I use, and that I feel adequate and comfortable to teach and to demonstrate.

It was then that it occurred to me that I was regularly using a form of augmented hypnosis in my 'Monday group'.

From there, I reflected on, if and how I have used it also in my individual sessions.

As if it was somehow ordained, that very same day, the 3rd of October 2017, I was presented with, not one, but two cases, where a session of hypnosis was clearly appropriate.

Not only that, but the use of an external aid became totally obvious; for the 1st case before I began, but for the 2nd, it only became clear, some ways in.

- For your interest, and to further explain some of the indications and uses of external aids, I will describe, in some detail, these two sessions, in the section on; 'uses of augmented hypnosis in individual sessions.'

So what do you mean by external aids?

Although not totally limited to; I would say, generally, other sounds, (music, drumming, singing, humming, chanting), using objects and getting the patient to move.

However, the use of incense and fragrant oils might also be interesting, (which are and have been used for centuries in various methods of cure).

And what are the uses and purposes of adding these elements?

The studies of how people learn have shown that different people have different channels of preference for acquiring and integrating information.

The main ones are; visual, auditive, and kinaesthetic, (linked to movement).

Although each person has their own preponderant choice, it has also been proven, that linking several of these, (multisensory learning), also greatly increases their capacity to understand and retain knowledge.

The Lexicon Reading Centre, suggest that;

"Multisensory teaching techniques and strategies stimulate learning by engaging students on multiple levels." They list four sensory input channels that can be activated; visual reasoning and learning, auditory techniques, tactile teaching methods and kinesthetic methods.[31]

Standard psychotherapeutic techniques, which is to say, talking, are directed, primarily at the cognitive function.

By accessing the patient's thinking process, we can often help them to reflect on, understand and even, open a space, for a new appreciation of their past, present and future experiences and behaviours.

Within this therapeutic space, the opening to certain personal truths, can, and often does, trigger blocked emotions, and can facilitate a strong emotional, cathartic experience.

---

[31] What is Multisensory Teaching Techniques?, https://www.lexiconreadingcenter.org/what-is-multisensory-teaching-techniques/ Retrieved 26.06.2019

However, we often find this approach blocked by strategic, intellectual defences, or the appreciation that the problem or its resolution, lies below the conscious functioning of the patient.

For those of use that have a training in a form of hypnotic technique, this is when we stop communicating directly with the patient's conscious mind and direct our attention towards the unconscious.

This can be effective in both unblocking certain memories, and, or releasing, imprisoned emotions.

However, even these techniques have their limitations, and it would be useful to find an extra added dimension, to support the therapeutic process, and reinforce integration of changes into their daily lives.

This is where the concept of augmented hypnosis comes in.

Talking therapy activates and directs itself towards the mind. (Auditive, Intellectual)

Hypnosis is an effective way to reach beyond the mind, and to reconnect to and release emotions. (Visual, Emotional)

Physical actions are directed towards the body functions, activating other sensory channels. (Kinaesthetic, Tactile).

By combining two or three channels, we can create a synergetic effect that multiplies the benefits of each separate approach.

Hence, the interest of these multisensorial, multichannel hypnotic techniques.

4. The oldest form of hypnosis

4.1 Discussion

This book is written to introduce you, the reader to the concept of augmented hypnosis.

However, I do not wish to give the impression that this is something that I have invented.

Quite the contrary, I am here to help you re-discover something that has existed since the dawn of time, and has continued to exist ever since, and that continues exist all around us.

The ultimate goal is to sensibilise therapists to this concept, so that they may, ultimately, integrate these ideas into their own practices, and hence, further help their patients and clients.

Just as I have deemed it useful and interesting to share an overview of the history of hypnosis, I would also like to reflect with you on the many forms of practice, that include the mechanisms of augmented hypnosis.

However, in many of these cases, there is one fundamental element missing, that of intention.

The difference between hypnosis and meditation and other similar psychological states is that, with hypnosis, there is a clearly defined intention behind the entering into a dissociated state, which does not exist in the same way in meditation.

However, when the intention is relaxation, or clearing the mind, the line becomes particularly unclear.

In fact, many, if not most of these experiences, would be more correctly defined as augmented meditations.

4.2 Trance dance, chanting & native drumming.

Many traditional cultures, where group rituals still take place, continue to create a trance state through repetitive dances, chanting and following the rhythm of a beating drum.

As these traditions have been handed down from generation to generation, it would be reasonable to suggest that these practices have remained, largely unchanged since time immemorial.

The most basic elements of a hypnotic induction are clearly present;
- a continual, strong, repetitive, outside stimulus
- that the stimulus continues for quite some time
- that the attention of the participant redirects from the outside towards an inner experience – which is to say, they dissociate.

4.3 Religious prayer and singing, (ecstatic states)

Ecstatic religious states could well be considered to be the natural continuation of the traditional ritual experience.

Depending on the specific religious practice, we can see how the two forms of experience meet. This is especially strong where the Christian church has been added over the traditional African culture and practices.

In certain church settings it is fairly easy to see the intention and support to enter into a secondary state, even leading onto intense religious ecstatic experiences.

However, this is not at all only specific to Christianity, one finds, for instance, in the Jewish tradition, something analogous with the rhythmic 'bobbing' of the religious Jews while 'davening'. Once the prayers are learned to point where the repetition becomes automatic, they also enter into a form of trance state.

4.4 Tai Chi, Qi gong, active meditations, and meditative katas

Moving towards the East, we find many forms of 'active meditation' techniques.

Although the focus and intention are not always exactly the same, the basics definitely are.

The student learns a number of very specific movements, these movements they then repeat, and repeat and repeat.

The focus of all their attention is on these repetitive actions.

Their consciousness is directed totally into the exactitude of movement.

In Tai Chi and Qi gong, there is the added suggestion, linked to the name of the movement, that invokes the image and the energy that they are reproducing.

Qi gong:

1. Turning the Prayer Wheel
2. Rotating the Knees
3. Crossed Arm Rotation
4. Picking Fruit
5. Swinging the Leg
6. Leg Bounce
7. Retreat and Advance
8. Grinding Corn
9. Polishing the Mirror

Tai Chi:

1 Part the wild horse's mane
2 The white crane spreads its wings
3 Grasp the bird's tail
4 Wave hands like clouds
5 High pat on the horse
6 Needle at sea bottom

Some of the main principles of Qi gong are:[32]

- Intentional movement: careful, flowing balanced style
- Rhythmic breathing: slow, deep, coordinated with fluid movement
- Awareness: calm, focused meditative state
- Visualization: of qi flow, philosophical tenets, aesthetics
- Chanting/Sound: use of sound as a focal point

For Tai Chi:[33]

"A Tai Chi form also begins with Stillness (Wu Chi), moves to the extremes of yin and yang in a flowing tide of continuous motion and comes back to stillness. An internal stillness is retained throughout the movements of the form. Meditation resting in the state of Wu Chi can bring peace of mind, serenity and greater wisdom."

---

[32] https://en.wikipedia.org/wiki/Qigong retrieved 08 10 2017
[33] http://www.yiheyuan.co.uk/Pages/TaiChiPhilosophy.aspx retrieved 08 10 2017

4.5 Yoga

Yoga is clearly a close cousin of the group of practices listed above, however, more firmly rooted in stillness, it deserves a special section of its own.

Yoga, especially hatha yoga, with its strong emphasis on the breath, allows for deep trance states within each of the poses.

Each pose offers the participant the opportunity to focus on a fixed point, long enough to integrate that as a none evolving sensorial stimulus, hence allowing for refocusing of the attention inwards, and the entering of the trance state.

4.6 Emotionally charged music

Listening to music and letting our attention wander, can also be considered a form of trance state.

This differs from the ritual, rhythmic, repetitive music that we mentioned above, as it is not due to the narrowing down of the stimulus to a boring and monotonous input.

Quite the contrary, the stimulus is interesting and varies. However, in the case where the listener is not offered, or not interested in the visual stimulation of watching the musicians play, then the visual field is not stimulated.

Even though the auditive senses are interested and active, without interesting visual input, the eyes tend to close, and from there, it is but a short step into dissociation.

4.7 Playing music

This is a most particular form of trance state, as the musician needs to be highly present, at some level, to play their instrument, and to remember the music that they are playing.

47

Hence, this is likely to happen, mostly, to only quite accomplished musicians.

Skilled players, after they have totally learned a piece, have integrated all the notes into some place of their psyche, and no longer have to think about them.

They would also needs have mastered the mechanics of playing it.

At this point, when the intellectual process of learning the notes is acquired, as is the physical dimension of actually playing the piece.

Then they can pass over to losing themselves in the emotional experience of playing it.

In this moment, they are both here, and elsewhere.

4.8 Singing and Dancing

In the same fashion that a musician can lose themselves in their playing, people can also lose themselves singing and dancing.

Again, this needs be differentiated from the more tribal experience of chanting and repetitive dance movements, as here we are talking about non-repetitive singing and more complex dance moves.

That is not to say that there cannot be situations where the song is based on simple repeated phrases and a basic melody, or that the dance steps are very easy to master and are repeated.

Only that it can also include quite complex song lyrics and structure, the same for possible complexities of the dance.

Likewise, a high level of mastery is necessary, so as to liberate the mind and the body from having to focus on the mechanics.

Hence allowing for the body to relax, (even when doing active and complex things), and releasing part of the mind to experience other things, even while directing these actions.

5 Inductions

5.1 Introduction to this section.

As explained in chapter 2, the main element used to induce a trance state is to install a constant, monotonous sensorial stimulus.

In modern hypnotic techniques, the main constant, monotonous sensorial stimulus is that of the voice of the hypnotist.

However, many hypnotists and hypnotherapists still use, for a variety of reasons; personal, patient orientated and, or linked to their specific therapeutic training, other means of inducing this most particular state.

Many of these induction techniques benefit from some external support, which brings them into the area of augmented hypnosis.

5.2 The 'EMDR induction'

EMDR, (**Eye Movement Desensitization and Reprocessing**), created by **Francine Shapiro** towards the end of the 1980's, is a respected treatment in the field of trauma and PTSD, (**Post Traumatic Stress Disorder**).[34]

It has a very clear and well-defined set of protocols that support clinicians in their treatments.

Not being one for clear and well-defined sets of protocols, I tend to fabricate my own approaches and techniques.

However, the very beginning of their protocol, benefits from a technique known as **alternating bilateral stimulation (ABS).**

Alternating bilateral stimulation was not discovered by Shapiro, nor any members of her team.

---

[34] History of EMDR https://www.emdr.com/history-of-emdr/ retrieved on the 02.06.2019

However, they strongly advance the benefits of ABS as an effective technique to aid relaxation.

On researching the subject, we find that the relaxing effects of alternating bilateral stimulation, have been known for centuries.

"**Unilateral forced nostril breathing (UFNB)**, a subset of yogic breathing (**pranayam**) techniques that were discovered/devised more than 5000 years ago. [includes …] the phenomenon called the "**nasal cycle**" (**NC**). In 1895

[**Richard**] **Kayser** was the first western scientist to document the NC. [Sentences re-ordered by the author]"[35]

---

[35] "Unilateral forced nostril breathing" Basic Science, Clinical Trials,and Selected Advanced Techniques
By David S. Shannahoff-Khalsa.
http://journals.sfu.ca/seemj/index.php/seemj/article/view/323
retrieved on the 02.06.2019

If one then links the following information:

"**Nadi shodhana**, or alternate nostril breathing, has a long history in **Ayurvedic medicine** and yoga, where it's thought to harmonize the two hemispheres of the brain.

"[36] [O]ne can easily arrive at the hypotheses that ABS succeeds to stimulate both sides of the brain and helps in relaxing the patient.

In my own reflection, alternatively stimulating the two hemispheres of the brain can have a positive effect.

Not only in facilitating relaxation, but also in dealing with trauma, especially when linked to a process that specifically directs the patient into that context.

---

[36] Yogis ahead of science: One nostril breathing determines how you feel. The Yoga Space
https://theyogaspace.co.uk/blog/PostId/261/yogis-ahead-of-science-one-nostril-breathing-determines-how-you-feel
retrieved on the 02.06.2019

(For a reflection on how ABS and the linking of left and right hemispheres might facilitate the treatment of trauma see A hypothesis on the effectiveness of EMDR in the appendix)

The EMDR protocol suggests using one's hand and arm to design an arc movement in front of the patient's face.

The fingers create a form of inverted pendulum which the patient follows with their eyes, (not the head). The moving of the eyes, and the changing of focus between them create the alternating bilateral stimulation.

I use this to start certain sessions. I then move my hand so that the patient looks up, at the same moment breathing deeply in. They hold their breath a short moment, and then slowly exhale, as I gently lower my hand, and as they follow the downward movement, their eyes naturally close.

5.3 Hypnotic induction using a pendulum

A hypnotist using a pendulum, or more often, a pocket watch, is the classical image that many people have of how a patient is led into the trance state.

The logic is exactly the same as that of the 'EMDR Induction'.

The constant, monotonous sensorial stimulus and the relaxing effect of the alternating bilateral stimulation are a perfect combination to induce a trance state.

Using either a pendulum, pocket watch, or one's fingers also allows for the therapist to tailor the amplitude, rhythm and motion, (arc, inverted arc, straight line, or wave), to the specific session and patient.

This freedom within the moment of the induction can be most useful.

5.4 Humming

I have recently introduced humming, (almost unconsciously), intertwined with hypnotic suggestions while using 'my' EMDR inspired induction technique'.

The speed, vibration and tonality, I find can add an extra dimension to the strength of the induction.

5.5 Beating the Drum

The drum in some form or other has been used to produce altered states of consciousness since the stone age.

"Artistic motifs at a number of late Neolithic megalithic ceremonial complexes in northern and western Europe (approximately 4000-2000 BCE) are thought to have been derived from entoptic hallucinatory imagery. I rish passage tombs or dolmen such as the site of Knowth, County Meath, are likely to have been designed as "multisensorial experiences" in which darkness and acoustic resonance could produce altered states of consciousness." [37]

Using a drumbeat to induce a trace state has been used world-over and since time immemorial in traditional, Shamanic cultures.

"**Shamanic drumming** is a form of drumming that serves to induce an altered state of awareness in its practitioner. It is believed that via the trance states that it produces, reality's spiritual dimension or "spirit world" can be accessed."[38]

---

[37] Altered States of Consciousness Carol R. Ember, Christina Carolus. HUMAN RELATIONS AREA FILES, https://hraf.yale.edu/ehc/summaries/altered-states-of-consciousness retrieved on the 02.06.2019

[38] Shamanic Drumming – Transforming our Lives with Vibration, Eagleshaman.com https://www.eagleshaman.com/shamanism/shamanic-drumming retrieved on the 08.06.2019

There some controversy over whether the shamanic journeying state is identical to that of a hypnotic trace, and whether the journey is nothing more than a (partly) guided hypnotic induction, here, is not the place to enter into this reflection.

[Although from extensive personal experience of both, I do believe that there are clear differences.]

What I would suggest is that the specific circumstances and intention of the person focalising the session, be it a shaman within the setting of a shamanic ritual or a therapist within their consultation, might have an important influence on the participant's experience.

With that vision clear in my mind, I have undertaken hypnotic sessions, simply clapping out a rhythm to enter the patient into a trace state and to accompany them in their process.

The specific benefit of this approach is that, without injecting myself into a situation where the patient needs to experience something 'alone', they still have the safety of a continual contact with me.

5.6 Silence

Michael Yapko, in his most interesting book on hypnosis, *"Essentials of Hypnosis"[39]*, has a specific section on the use of silence in trancework.

"Silence can be a useful deepening technique if used skilfully."

However, if one wishes to bother to undertake a 'Google Search', one can find many other hypnotherapists that have come to the same conclusion.

---

[39] Michael Yapko Routledge; *Essentials of Hypnosis*, 2 edition (October 15, 2014)

As with many things, I tend to take usual techniques and extend them a little further.

My use of silence is a standard part of my therapeutic approach, which I use very often in my inductions.

However, I tend to include between five and ten minutes in some sessions, depending on the type and indication of and for hypnosis that I am undertaking.

In many sessions I use my EMDR inspired induction and I continue talking, offering the patient the opportunity to continually deepen the trance, all the while inviting the deepest parts of the person to seek out and deal with whatever the particular problem might be.

Within this stage, the patient can, if they feel motivated, share with me any experiences or memories that they are experiencing.

However, if after 20 to 30 minutes they still have not felt to interact, I then more or less stop talking and leave them 'to go deeper' in silence.

I interject, from time to time, a phrase that reinforces the message but nothing more.

However, if I notice that the patient is having a clear reaction to something, then I will ask what is happening and if they wish to express it.

Obviously if they choose to share these experiences, then an interactive exchange then takes place and I work with that.

It should be noted that I am happy to leave sessions with no interaction with the patient, if that is what works for them in the moment,

As, for me, the goal of hypnosis is to contact the unconscious, inaccessible parts of the psyche.

It might be much less 'rewarding' for both the patient and the therapist to have sessions where there might be no reaction, in the moment.

However, for the patient, the subtle, organic changes that follow, (sometimes several weeks after the session(s)), are natural and much more robust than the exciting, impressive cathartic abreactions that one often sees in films and TV.

(Not that don't have and appreciate cathartic sessions!)

Hence, silence is an important part of my hypnotic techniques.

5.7 The Pinch

This is one of my favourite inductions.

The pinch is often taught, by me, as an induction of preference for those that wish to learn self or autohypnosis.

Not only this, but it possibly the only generally used form of trance that people can use to calm themselves while still being active in their daily lives.

In fact, I teach this to my patients to help them calm themselves down in situations of public speaking or exams.

For a more complete discussion on the uses of this induction and trance state, I have added some extra sections at the end of this work.

What is important to note here is that this practice serves both as an induction and as an anchor.

The technique in itself is quite simple to understand and to do.

The patient consciously presses, on either one or both hands, the thumb and index fingers together, in such a way to produce the greatest area of contact possible.

They then play with the pressure between the thumb and index, noting the sensation(s) that this creates.

By focusing on these, we recreate, to some degree, induced by the patient themselves, the constant, monotonous sensorial stimulus, and yet not.

Before continuing, I will need to take a short moment to share my vision of teaching in general and by extension teaching autohypnosis.

I am a convinced disciple in the theories of child development of **Lev Vygotsky** (1896 –1934).

Vygotsky's fundamental vision of learning is that it is strongly supported by an outside supporting teacher.

"Vygotsky states cognitive development stems from social interactions from guided learning within the **zone of proximal development** as children and their partner's co-construct knowledge."[40]

My approach is to first 'do' for the other, (usually one of my children). Then I involve them to a limited degree in the operation.

From there on, they take over more and more of the task. Until finally my role is simply to validate their acquisition of their new competence.

In the same vein, and coherent with many other practitioners, I teach autohypnosis as a continuation from hetero-hypnosis.

---

[40] Lev Vygotsky – Simply Psychology
https://www.simplypsychology.org/vygotsky.html retrieved on the 09.06.2019

"Most clinicians teach self-hypnosis through hetero-hypnosis, in part by direct or indirect posthypnotic suggestion

. ...According to the present author, self-hypnosis taught through hetero-hypnotic experiences is effective as a method for physical and emotional tranquilization in nearly all subjects."[41]

To return to the subject in question, the induction through the pinch.

Although this is mostly taught as a self-hypnotic induction, I always start by leading as if it is a regular hypnotic session.

I explain the concept and invite the patient to choose which hand, or to use both hands.

---

[41] Teaching self-hypnosis to adults, Paul Sacerdote International Journal of Clinical and Experimental Hypnosis Volume 29, 1981 - Issue 3 https://www.tandfonline.com/doi/abs/10.1080/002071481084 09162 retrieved on the 09.06.2019

Then to press the thumb(s) and index together, contacting the pulpy parts, so as have the greatest area of contact possible.

They are then asked to focus on the sensations that they are feeling; heat, coolness, attraction, repulsion, vibrations, tickling, feeling that the fingers are stuck together, or melting into each other, or possibly with the right amount of pressure, that they might even feel their own heartbeat.

I also suggest that they also, in parallel notice their breathing, which, 'naturally' is beginning to become deeper and slower.

In this, first experience of the pinch, I finally suggest that their eyes are likely to be feeling heavy and that they might feel more comfortable if they let them close.

I continue to help them focalise on the experiences of the contact between them and themselves, and then to allow themselves to go deeper and deeper into the experience.

I then pass a relatively long moment in silence, which, as explained above, I find greatly reinforces to trance experience.

After some moments I inform the patient that in a moment I will instruct them to open their eyes, but they are to remain calm and not to speak.

I then instruct them to open their eyes and then immediately to, themselves, return into the trance state.

I gently continue to coach them, from time to time, to focus on the sensations linked to the contact of their fingers, but only as if to remind them of the process.

They easily slip back into the trance state and when reawakened have the satisfaction of having led themselves into a trance.

If there remains enough time, I will support them in returning a third time into the trance.

The reason why I instruct them to remain calm and not to speak after coming out of the first trance, is create a condition that we call fractionation.

By entering, exiting and re-entering into a trance, the trance state becomes deeper each time.

By using fractionation, the patient, with only minimum help from me, easily enters a deep and satisfying trance, re-enforcing their experience and their confidence.

5.8 'Jeans'

This is another induction based on physical sensations.

This is not an induction that I use much, but as it clearly enters into the subject area, I have thought to include it.

[Of course, the patient does not have to be wearing jeans, it is just an easy way to think if this technique.]

This can be particularly useful for patients that seem to lack the patience or the ability to focus long enough on the 'constant, monotonous sensorial stimulus' to succeed to enter into the trance state.

The patient is invited to place their hands flat on their laps, (palms down). They are then instructed to focus their attention to the feel of the texture of their clothes.

Are they smooth, rough, warm, cold, hard, soft...?

Again, the patient is active in the process, but yet is still directed to focus on a stimulus that vastly narrows their field of awareness, and eventually becomes monotonous.

And so enter into the trance …

5.9 The Thumb

This is a 'pure' autohypnotic technique.

Again, this is not a technique that I have used recently, but as it also fits within the concept of augmented hypnosis, I have thought to include it.

The process of first leading the patient into the trace, fractionating and getting them to re-enter into the trance, is identical.

The technique is in itself easy enough to explain.

They lift up one of their arms in front of them, (palm facing downwards), so that their hand is at the same level as their eyes.

They close their hand into a fist, (as if hitching for a ride), but with their thumb sticking out horizontally.

They then fix their attention on their thumb, (any part; the articulation, the half moon of the nail, or the tip of the nail itself).

'By itself, the arm will begin to descend.' (It is most important to use the 'body-subject language' as it re-enforces the body experience and reduces the cognitive activity).

'At its own speed, as it chooses'. The patient is instructed to follow the descent of their thumb with their eyes, while keeping their head stationary.

'You might notice that your breathing becomes slower and deeper'. (A suggestion linked to the change in the patient's breathing is often helpful, but not essential).

'Eventually your hand will descend onto your lap and by then your eyes will have closed, and you will find yourself in a relaxed, peaceful state.'

And so it is …

6 Individual Sessions

6.1 Introduction to Individual Sessions

Individual sessions of hypnosis are the most usual and standard settings that the hypnotherapist will find themselves in.

Although there are more than a few similar techniques; guided meditation, sophrology etc., that are close 'cousins', yet different, they still, generally, limit themselves to simply speaking to the patient / client.

The individual sessions that I will describe below all, in some way or other benefit from the extra something that augmented hypnosis uses to reinforce the hypnotic process.

Nb. For the sake of simplicity, and following a usual tendency, I will refer to these hypnotic processes as inductions,

Even though technically speaking an induction is the leading into the trance state and not the session itself.

6.2 The flower

The flower is an induction close to my heart. I used it, (maybe even created it), during my wife's first pregnancy.

Quite early on in the pregnancy she started having strong and potentially dangerous, (for our baby), contractions and so we used this, for quite some time, on an almost daily basis.

I have included most of the chapter from my book, 'Remember' in the Annexes, in which I treat this induction quite fully.

Hence, I will limit the information in this section to the minimum.

This induction can have several indications; releasing tension, (physical, mental, emotional), opening up to new experiences, even specifically opening to female sexuality.

The instructions to the patient are more than simple:

'For this exercise allow your hand or hands to close into a quite tight fist.
During this induction your hand or hands can open more and more, following the course of the opening of the flower. '

The induction follows the course of a half day, where the flower, first tightly shut, slowly and gently opens more and more as the light and warmth of the sun increase until it reaches its zenith.

As I speak of the petals beginning to relax and to open, I also suggest the patient's fingers relax and open.

Which, of course, they do …

6.3 Draining out the tension / poison

This induction although in some aspects is similar to the Flower, has a most interesting functioning.

The concept, as with most inductions, is simple and easy to explain.

'In your hand is a ball of tissues.

Tissues are used to absorb stuff that we wish to dispose of.

Within yourself you have stuff that is not good for you to keep.

During this session your body, emotions, and, or mind will allow the tissues to absorb some of this stuff that you would be better off without.

At some point, when it feels that the tissues have absorbed as much as seems appropriate for now, your hand will choose to open, and the tissues will fall onto the floor.

All that has been absorbed by the tissues will then be released from you.'

6.4 Pulling out thorns

This induction is based on a single and unusual incident, however I have thought to add it to illustrate the necessity of the hypnotist to remain open and creative during every session.

I was leading a session in which the patient was complaining about a painful relationship that they were in but couldn't find a way to remove herself from it.

That very morning I had decided that the cactus plant in my office had become impossibly big and invasive of the space, so I had decided to cut it down.

As I had bought it when moving into my office, I was loth just to chop it down and throw it away.

So I cut a number of fronds, ('leaves') and placed them in water so that they might regrow. [Which quite a few have Ed.]

Confronted with the patient's blockage, and her own imagery. I had the inspiration to use one of the smaller and less prickly fronds.

With the permission of the patient I carefully placed it in her hand and directed her to press it gently onto her chest.

I then linked her experience of having this painful relationship with the pricking sensation of the cactus and allowed her to make the choice to remove it.

The effect was clearly much, much stronger than a classic induction could ever have been.

6.5 Breaking the bonds

This is an interesting induction but takes a minimum of preparation.

What seems to work best is using two sheets of kitchen paper towels, still joined by the perforations.

The patient is invited, before the induction begins to grab one end of each of the towels in each of their hands.

During the induction, I refer to a situation in which they feel bound and suggest that they gently pull on the towels until they experience their movement limited by them.

I then suggest that, in fact they do have the means to free themselves, if only they would give themselves permission to use this inner force.

When I feel that they are sufficiently motivated, I allow them to release their power and break their bonds.

The paper rips into two, and they are freed!

6.6 Energy Transfer

This is an induction that I use for very specific cases when the patient is so low, sad, depressed that there is a great need for an immediate boost.

Also, because it implies a physical contact between the therapist and the patient, one must be sure that the patient is totally comfortable with such a contact while in the particularly vulnerable state of trance.

There is also the question of the patient's belief system. If they are open to the idea that the therapist can channel positive energy through him / herself into the patient, then this can be a useful induction.

It would go without saying that the therapist must also be open to such a concept.

Before or just after leading the patient into a trance state, the therapist takes the patient's hand.

The therapist then suggests that they will open themselves to 'universal energy', (or whatever works for them), and that energy will flow through them, down their arm, into their hand and finally into the patient.

That the patient will feel something; heat, vibrations, pressure, etc., which will be their way of experiencing the energy flowing in.

From there one continues to reinforce the benefits of this; healing, energising, calming, etc., energy.

The concept can even be further developed to include the patient sending out some of this positive energy to someone in need of help and support.

Admittedly this intervention could be seen as crossing the boundaries of therapy and entering into the worlds of Shamanism or even Magic.

As to be expected, some therapists or patients can certainly feel uncomfortable with this.

However, whether or not there is any proof that the infusion of energy is a reality that exists or is just a psychological construct in the minds of the therapist and the patient, I have certainly seen the benefit of such an intervention.

7 Couple Sessions

7.1 Introduction to Couple Sessions

As one might imagine, it is rather rare to use hypnosis in a couple setting.

However, it is not totally unknown to me, and they usually include the extra dimension that augmented hypnosis offers.

As one might image, I mostly see couples to deal with communication and relationship issues.

Although there are usually many practical aspects to deal with, the losing of trust and falling out of love, can be the hardest to overcome.

After many years of experience, I feel that I have developed a good sense of when a couple is likely to have a deep bond, even if they have 'lost contact' on the surface.

In these specific circumstances, I offer them this following induction…

7.2 Linking together

I have them sit fairly close together and lead them into a trance state. I talk of whatever seems appropriate for this couple, some of their shared, positive history.

I then talk about how tides rise and fall, how problems can come and go, but yet some things still and always remain.

I talk about the deep connection that they still have for each other, and I then invite them to hold hands.

'Feel the warmth, feel the energy between you.'

I invite them to go deeply into their own feelings, their own contact with themselves and that deep contact with their partner.

As often, I leave a long moment of silence, which since there is no other interesting stimulus, attracts them to invest even more in the only one 'to hand'.

8 Group Sessions

8.1 Introduction to Group Sessions

In 2010 my wife, (a state registered psychiatrist and psychotherapist), and I founded a group practice, 'D'un Monde à l'Autre', (from one world to the next), to work with immigrants in a transcultural setting.

One of major advantages of working with other therapists was that we were able to rent part of a beautiful building, in the centre of Lausanne.

A building that also boasted a large space that we have been able to use as a group therapy room.

For most of the last nine years, I have been running groups, on different themes, but with one underlying thread, accessing the hidden resources through indirect means.

I start each session with a short discussion of the subject of the week, either suggested by one of the participants or something of my own inspiration.

I then lead them into a group trance where I invoke the image or energy that we will be working on.

From there, without bringing them fully out of the trance, they continue with a physical exercise, which offers them an active dimension of the same theme

After the exercise there is time to discuss and share their experiences. [And drink tea and munch biscuits Ed.]

The benefit of this threefold approach is that the emotional, (hypnosis), physical and mental channels are all integrated into one coherent session.

Here are a small sampling of these sessions.

8.2 Trust – Leading the blind

Lack of trust, confidence in ourselves or in those around us can leave us living in fear and isolation.

Opening up to trust is not simple nor obvious, however it is sometimes necessary so as to benefit from all that one can gain, if only one could learn to trust …

This is a classic trust exercise, used in many different workshops and settings.

The participants find themselves a partner, one of them is blindfolded while the other leads them around the room.

As there are other couples, and sometimes small objects, the people leading need to be most attentive that their 'blind' partner is kept safe from bumping into other people or things.

8.3 Rhino – vs Manipulation & Outside control

Timidity, social correctitude, uncertainty, poor self-image, lack of confidence, etc., can severely limit one's ability to push through the resistance of ourselves and others in the research of our goals.

In this exercise we line up all the participants, bar one, (the Rhino).

The Rhino's task is break through the wall of resistance and reach their ultimate goal.

We are fortunate to have found some solid square shaped cushions that we use for multiple purposes.

The members of the wall hold up their cushions at chest level as a protective shield.

The Rhino then slowly charges the wall, which does its best to block the passage through.

91

However, (using pressure but not violence), the Rhino always finally succeeds to push through line and to attain their goal.

8.4 Protection – I am the parent, I am the child

Many of us, but especially our patients have lacked adequate physical and, or emotional support during childhood. Bowlby's Attachment Theory,[42] elegantly argues for the importance of 'holding' in early childhood and the damage that the lack thereof can have on the emotional development of the person.

The feeling of not being protected, nor the ability to protect others is a common theme amongst fragile populations.

---

[42] The origins of attachment theory: John Bowlby and Mary Ainsworth. Bretherton, Inge Developmental Psychology, Vol 28(5), Sep 1992, 759-775
https://psycnet.apa.org/doiLanding?doi=10.1037%2F0012-1649.28.5.759   retrieved on the 11.06.2019

This session was created to respond towards helping those with such problems.

The patients are given a soft pillow to hug during the induction moment.

I then regress them back to their earliest childhood and split them between being, at the same time the baby being held, and the parent that is holding them.

They then get up and walk around the space, caring and protecting themselves: the baby.

At the same time expressing openness and care towards the other participants, creating the experience of a global, protected space.

(Soft music can also add to the generally womb-like ambience.)

From time to time I gently remind them that they are both the baby; loved, supported and protected, and also the kind, loving, strong protector.

8.5 Tree – & Bendy Tree

Strength, flexibility and solidity, both mental and emotional are important assets to have if we are to succeed to cope with the challenges of modern life.

Unfortunately, when we are not functioning well, we have a tendency to become mentally and emotionally rigid. And; either like an old, dry branch, brittle and easily breakable, or a sick tree with weakened roots, ready to be blown down by the first storms of Autumn, we are in constant danger from our environment.

This session was devised to counter the natural tendencies of weak, rigid defensive reactions that my patients in difficulty would reactively seek out in moments of stress.

In this induction, for which the participants are standing, feet slightly apart, I would invoke the idea of their walking in a forest, finding a tree that they were attracted to a make contact with it.

94

Then to hug the tree, and finally to merge with it.

I direct them to focus on their legs and then feet and then their toes. As the tree they can feel their roots reaching deep, deep down into the rich, safe and welcoming earth. The deeper they allow their consciousnesses to delve the more they experience being nourished and anchored by the Mother Earth.

From there, I invite them to allow their attention to raise upwards, while still holding an awareness on the feeling of being solidly planted into the ground.

To rise upwards, through the roots, into the trunk and then the intricate network of their branches.

I then invoke a breeze, gentle and light, they feel the wind, but it hardly affects them.

Then the wind increases its power, they start to gently sway.

And as the storm approaches, I remind them of how solidly they are implanted into the ground. Their tree-selves bend and sway with the wind.

He is their dance partner, he leads them, they, solid on their contact with the ground, respond to the impetus of the storm.

They flow with the movement, it is exciting, thrilling, intense.

Finally, the storm subsides, tired but satisfied they relax…

8.6 Energy, Fire – Wing Chung Punch

We all have moments when we feel weak, tired and have difficulty energising and protecting ourselves.

There is also, often, a resistance again expressing powerful, 'negative' emotions.

Many traditions speak of the Hara Centre or the Solar Plexus, (around the belly button), as the central energy point of the body.

And that by focusing on it, it is possible to increase the body's energy level.

As a teenager I studied a little of Kung Fu. The Wing Chung punch is part of that discipline.

The Wing Chung punch is interesting in that it is a circular movement; with one arm sliding over the other, punching and then, while withdrawing, sliding under the other arm, which is starting its own punching motion.

Which means that it lends itself particularly well as a form of active meditation.

The speed and the force depend on the will and desire of the participant. However, it is important to push them into entering into the spirit of the exercise.

The induction speaks of the energy and power that we have available within ourselves, only we need to learn how to contact it and release its potent force.

And how our education is to not allow ourselves to contact what is often mistaken as anger or violence.

The participants are then invited to practice the punch with all the psychical and emotional energy that they can find within themselves. The using of the voice to reinforce the action is strongly supported.

8.7 Through the tunnel of despair

To feel that one's life is blocked and there is way to advance, that there is no future is one of the most often found symptoms of depression.

Not that one needs to be clinically depressed to have these feelings; we all are likely to have them from time to time.

For my group, I focus my induction on the image of advancing through the darkness, no matter how difficult or scary that it might seem, to finally emerge into the success of the light.

For a physical experience to reinforce this story, I took a blanket which placed on the floor held in place by some of participants.

One by one, each member of the group was invited to crawl through this 'tunnel'. Being held down by the others, this was not without a certain challenge.

Before each person had their turn, I reinforced the message of how this was a difficult, even scary task and they needed to be brave and tenacious to be able to succeed.

Depending on the size, strength and psychologic state of each, I varied the difficulty of crawling through the blanket tunnel.

Which meant that each faced a real challenge, based on their own capacities, and that reaching the end was indeed a success in their own terms.

8.8 Perambulating pyramid – walking a narrow bridge with help to balance.

Strength and balance in many areas of our lives would always be useful. However, when people are psychologically unwell, these are often two of the elements that weaken significantly.

There are inductions that speak of strength and solidity; namely the Tree and the Mountain, (see above and below).

The limitations of those two inductions just mentioned is that they are stationary, and their strength is a result of either having strong roots deeply embedded in the earth or having such weight and mass that they cannot be assailed.

In our daily lives we need to be mobile, and yet solid enough to withstand the powerful winds of life's troubles and tribulations.

The image that I offer during the induction is that of a mobile pyramid.

To create an experience that will anchor such a reality I built a narrow bridge out of square cushions for the participants to walk along.

However, a pyramid is wider at the bottom than the top, which is what brings its stability.

To add such a dimension, we had two other members of the group walk along each side of the bridge, being a physical support and guaranteeing a balance that without would make the passage particularly difficult.

(A pile of cushions is not the most solid structure to walk across).

8.9 Get up!! – bent down pillow pressing on back

To be heavily weighed down by life's problems can happen to anyone, for our patients, already exhausted and fragilized by their sickness, they can seem ten times worse.

The induction sets the scene invoking the crushing weight of their problems and the Herculean effort needed to rise up and assume them.

The practical exercise is for the patients, in turn, to crouch down and to have our multipurpose square cushions piled onto their backs.

I hold the cushions in place and assert an extra pressure to assure that the patient needs to make a real effort to get up.

After allowing them to struggle long enough to feel the need to really push with all their force, they succeed to get back up onto their feet.

8.10 Being a mountain

This was one of the early sessions that we had, but as I have decided to finish with a person anecdote from one of my patients, I thought to leave it to the end.

A poor self-image and a susceptibility to both external and internal criticism leaves people particularly vulnerable to anguish and depression.

'I am who I am, and that's okay', is not an affirmation without possible negative connotations, but when the opposite is someone's truth, then this is an important position to be able to assume.

The mountain is heavy, solid, virtually permanent, impossible to move, in fact, almost impossible to affect in any way.

During the induction I suggested that the words and actions of others are no more than the wind and a small hammer tapping on the mountain's surface. In reality, they can do no real harm.

After the induction the participant, as often, protected with one of our famous, square cushions stands with their front foot facing forward and back foot at a ninety-degree angle to their body, a particularly solid stance.

Another participant attempts to then push the first one over. If the 'pusher' is bigger, stronger, heavier than the 'mountain', there could be a danger that they might succeed, but since I am standing behind the 'mountain', and I weigh over 95 kgs, (about 200 lbs), and I am leaning on their back as a physical support, there is never any risk of that occurring.

The week after we undertook this session, one of the participants shared with the group her experience from over the weekend.

So as to fully understand the value of this experience for my patient it is necessary for me to give some background details of her life.

[Certain details have been modified to protect her identity and respect the medical secret.]

The patient comes from a well-respected professional Spanish family. While studying at the University of Lausanne she met, fell in love with and eventually married a young lawyer from a very 'old' and wealthy Swiss family.

Notwithstanding that she is beautiful, intelligent and comes from a 'good family', her free, open, emotionally expressive personality and behaviours have never allowed her to be fully accepted by her, rather rigid and discreet Swiss family.

Clearly, to have fallen into quite an important depression, she also has certain fragilities linked to her early life experiences, but the current crisis has much to do with her feelings of inferiority due to her in-laws constant criticisms, and that no-one, (especially her husband), is here to defend her.

105

The choice to focus on the image of the mountain was mostly for her to strengthen her own ability to defend herself.

(As many of the participants of the groups are my own patients that I follow individually, or who's problems I am quite aware of, I often choose a theme that I know will be of particular use and interest for them.)

So this is what she shared with the group, the following week.

"I was sitting with my family Saturday evening; my husband, my in-laws and my two sons.

My father-in-law turns to me, smiling asked me how my job seeking was going.

Knowing full well that I am not in a state to look for work at the moment, this is pure sadism.

I started to feel both angry and upset.

Often in this type of situation I would either respond very aggressively, to which everyone would look shocked and surprised, or I would find some weak excuse to leave the table and go and cry in the kitchen.

As he was talking quite close to my face, I could feel his breath which then reminded me of the thing with the mountain.

So I stopped thinking about him, and weirdly even about me and concentrated of feeling like a mountain.

Strong, heavy and not affected by the inconsequential wind of his words.

After only a few seconds I began to feel much calmer. I turned back to him.

"Fine, so how are you enjoying not working anymore?"

As someone that had clearly invested too much of his time and energy in his profession, retirement was not that easy for him to benefit from.

I then turned to my oldest son and started a conversation about his new school project."

9 Hypno-flushing

9.1 Humaniversity Flushing – The Pure Experience

'Flushing' is a powerful emotional release technique developed at the Humaniversity by Veeresh.[43]

The Humaniversity website describes Flushing in these terms:[44]

"Flushing is a powerful process of emotional release and awareness. It takes you on an exciting journey to the core of your being.

---

[43] Veeresh born Denny Yuson-Sánchez in New York City in 1938. An ex heroin addict, founded in 1978 what is now known as the OSHO Humaniversity, an independent, residential personal development and training institute on the North Sea coast of the Netherlands.
https://www.humaniversity.com/veeresh retrieved on the 16.06.2019
[44] Humaniversity Flushing
https://www.feelyourbody.info/emotional-expression retrieved on the 16.06.2019

… In this workshop you will have many different opportunities to experience intense expression and supportive connections, and to re-discover your loving self.

You will come out empowered, feeling lighter, joyful and able to make positive changes in your life."

I had the incredible opportunity to participate in a weekend of Flushing, this particular workshop was led by the wonderful Geetee.

Clearly each participant will have their own different experiences and their own personal level of success.

Whatever the outcome, it is a powerful and well structured, cathartic experience.

I will describe the essential stages of this process, and the setting which is offered to facilitate the participants to succeed to enter into the necessary psychic states so that blocked emotions can be released.

- All other details are intentionally left in obscurity so as to leave interested future participants the opportunity to discover the full experience first-hand.

I also would presume that it would be totally obvious that one would not imagine to attempt to use the technique explained below without, at least, fully experiencing a complete Flushing workshop run by the Humaniversity professionals.

Also, as I have mentioned below, participants in the workshop will all succeed, to some level or other to go through the process.

Where-as, my own experiences with the technique have led to quite mixed results.

This process has four stages, "I Hate.", "No", "I have the Power" and "I Love".

Of course this is just one facet of the workshops which use this technique, and there are different variants and multiple sessions used by the focalisers.

The Humaniversity invites, (by my own estimation), 30 to 50 participants, plus they call on several of their own group leaders to lead the sessions and have between 10 to 20 helpers who support the group and its process.

Each stage lasts for quite a long time and the participants are strongly encouraged to deeply feel each emotion / position.

9.2 A personal reflection.

A personal reflection on a psychological interpretation of the process.

Depression and anxiety are two states that many if not most people experience at some level, quite often during their lives.

One way that I look at these is from an angle of how their energy is being expressed or not.

Sometimes we find ourselves in situations where something is not happening as we need it to, but other circumstances make it seem impossible to change.

For instance, we are having a difficult time at work but are afraid to demission because we need the job and don't have the confidence that we can find another.

There are certain dimensions of our energy that want to give in our notice but are blocked by other dimensions that stop ourselves from doing so.

Sometimes we are aware of this process, sometimes not. Not being aware is not a sign of mental disorder, it is a normal human mechanism.

This inner conflict, which I sometimes present to patients as the human equivalent of a country having a civil war, uses one block of our energy to frustrate another, leaving little spare for normal life.

Even an agriculturally rich country can find itself in a state of famine during a civil war.

The discomfort, sadness and lack of energy that comes from this is often the cause of what we experience as depression.

On the other hand, there are situations that have or might do us harm but to allow ourselves to be conscious of them would be, to us unthinkable or unacceptable.

The usual reactions to danger are flight, fight or freeze, (hiding). However, if we cannot accept a person or a situation as 'dangerous', then we deny ourselves these basic survival reactions and remain in a condition of high alert without the means to respond appropriately.

In these situations, our warning alarms continue to sound, we respond to false target after false target, as the real danger is hidden from view.

Our energy is continually but inappropriately being used.

These are the circumstances that create the awful condition of chronic anxiety.

Of course, life is much, much more complex, and multi-factorial. However, these heavily over-simplified examples, give a more accessible image of how one might understand these mechanisms.

The sadness and feeling of hopelessness in depression and the constant alertness towards small but potentially dangerous situations and experiences are, in reality, only ways to protect the person against a direct contact with feelings, thoughts and ideas that are even more upsetting.

Flushing is a process that begins by forcing the participant to break through these basic defences.

9.3 "I Hate"

"I Hate", directs the person's energy towards people, (including themselves) that, to some level, even slightly, have upset them.

And just as the hypnotic induction takes a single stimulus upon which they focus their attention to enter into the trance state, "I Hate" focalises their energy so to direct it into a single energy flow.

This flow eventually overrides the resistance to negative expression in the depressive position and allows them to direct their anger towards the 'unacceptable' target in the anxious one.

Once the energy has been liberated and directed, one can move onto the 2nd step.

9.4 "No"

 "No", is the ultimate defence, the unassailable barrier.

Once their energy has become freely available, the first and most important use is to able to defend themselves.

It is from behind this wall, in the moment of safety that they can start to relax, to repair, to reinforce their energy and their confidence in themselves.

It is also a position from which that one does not need to attack, to hurt or to destroy, to feel that one is able to survive.

9.5 "I have the Power"

"I have the Power". This is the logical next step in the evolving ascension towards increasing power and confidence.

From the bastion of their impenetrable wall of energy, they can now marshal their resources and redirect their energy into a powerful field of 'will'.

There is no more need for violence, nor does one have to depend on defence, the confidence of the use of their energy to control people and their environment is enough.

9.6 "I Love"

"I Love", is the ultimate expression of energy. When there is no more danger or threat, when one has the confidence that one can help or harm the other at will, then acceptance and forgiveness are all that the energy has left to do.

9.7 Hypno – Flushing

Having gone through and benefited from the experience myself, when I came across certain of my patients that I estimated might also benefit from such an approach I mentioned this workshop as a possibility.

However, being;
a) Francophone,
b) Not into New-Age therapies,
and c) not particularly motivated to spend the time and money necessary, there were no 'takers'.

Still feeling that such an experience could be of use, I then reflected on how I might offer something resembling the Humaniversity Flushing within the confines and limitations of my practice.

The 'solution' was the creation of Hypno-flushing.

9.8 The Context

The first thing to consider is that we are working in a usual clinical setting, the rich and complex infrastructure of the Humaniversity is not available to us.

Hence there are several considerations to take into account:

In general, one is limited to the length of each therapy session.

One is also limited to how much noise one can comfortably make.

As it is essential that the process can take the time necessary to reach its natural conclusion, I always program the session at the end of the day and clear my evening. (Between two to three hours is reasonable to budget, but one needs to stay flexible!)

Clearly there is likely to be a practical question of 'billing'. Most health insurances limit sessions to one to one and a half hours.

This is a facture to clarify with the patient before advancing any further.

For myself, I choose to bill the insurance at the maximum that they will allow and offer any additional time taken freely to the patient.

On the question of noise, this depends very much on the situation of your workplace.

By programming the session at the end of the working day, there is more chance that, in a professional environment, everyone else has finished for the day, and noise is less of a problem.

However, if there are likely to be neighbours who will be disturbed by the patient screaming, I start off with teaching them a technique that I have named, 'the silent scream'.

9.9 The Silent Scream

One might have watched an old vampire movie where the vampire makes a strange hissing, screaming sound.

They open their mouths fully, make a kind of 'haaa' sound that is carried by the expulsion of air, yet the vocal cords seem to not vibrate.

This is quite easy to replicate, and one can express a strong emotion, yet remain, more or less silent.

9.10 The Sessions

To give a reasonable view of how this type of intervention can happen, I have decided to document my first three experiences of using this technique as well as the reactions of the patients.

9.11 P1

P1.   I was working in office space that I
only rented the one room, I could not
assume that there would not be other people
in the building, even in the evening. Hence,
I began the session teaching and practicing
the 'silent scream' with the patient.

After this was comfortably in place I started
with a general induction, allowing the
patient to relax and open up to the next
steps.

"I Hate". I then introduced the concept of a
volcano that had been waiting to erupt for a
long time. We repeated, 'I hate', for a long
moment until he started spontaneously
adding names of people that he needed to
target.

"No". I followed this with the idea of
constructing a barrier, which followed
naturally on.

123

"I have the power". From here on, I only needed to suggest the next steps, and he easily found this energy.

"I love". This was very deep and quiet.

The patient completed the session, relaxed, smiling and appreciative.

However, I had no further feedback as I haven't seen the patient since!

9.12 P2

P2.   We started with a general relaxation and then introduced the 'silent scream' which went well.

"I Hate". This began with some difficulty, beating a pillow seemed to help, but yet I wasn't convinced.

We tried standing up, we tried with him punching and yet I continued to have the feeling that he wasn't really 'committed'.

124

After less than an hour I chose to end the experiment as I could see that we were not succeeding to break through his psychological defences.

My later reflection was that maybe he was 'too fragile' for this type of intervention. However, he expressed that he still found the session of value and in his future sessions often referred to it as a positive experience.

9.13 P3

P3.   We started with silent scream, but he didn't succeed well with it.
So we tried again with a clear 'HA', sound and movement while standing.

After a moment, the patient stopped the process, "I'm not into it, I'm watching myself doing it."

We took a moment to discuss the concept and benefit of the watcher, I then valorised its function.

We then restarted the 'HA', this time it worked better.

"I Hate". We continued standing, and from my point of view, he seemed to be entering into the process, until he stopped again.

"I'm not in it."

So we started again, this time it continued and worked well.

"No". Good, nothing special

"I Have the Power". To begin with, I was concerned that nothing seemed to be happening. Then I noticed that he was gently humming.

I invited him to increase what he was doing, and that was the moment that he started to sing.

126

"I Love". After the singing, in the 'power' section, it was natural to continue into the final stage.

The next session brought a different person into my consultation. He seemed taller, surely much more positive, much more confident.

Someone that had often experienced others taking advantage of him was more than happy to share with me the events of one week.

Not only had he succeed to land an excellent job with great conditions, but someone who he had helped in the past had suddenly decided to thank him by sending him a brand-new computer.

It would be highly improbable that these two events could have anything to do with the hypno-flushing, but it was a particularly useful coincidence, just the same.

9.14 Nothing new under the sun

While generally researching this book, I have accidently come across a paper that joins both a silent technique and a cathartic release of anger and other phases that have interesting similarities to hypno-flushing.

For those that might be interested to investigate further, one might well benefit to read of *The Therapeutic Release of Anger*: Helen Watkins's Silent Abreaction and Subsequent Elaborations of the Anger Rock[45]

---

[45] The Therapeutic Release of Anger: Helen Watkins's Silent Abreaction and Subsequent Elaborations of the Anger Rock Intl. Journal of Clinical and Experimental Hypnosis, 57(1): 47–63, 2009 Copyright © International Journal of Clinical and Experimental Hypnosis ISSN: 0020-7144 print / 1744-5183 online DOI: 10.1080/00207140802463633 https://www.academia.edu/4700835/The_Therapeutic_Releas e_of_Anger_Helen_Watkinss_Silent_Abreaction_and_Subseq uent_Elaborations_of_the_Anger_Rock Retrieved the 24.06.2019

10 Integrating with Equine Assisted Therapy.

10.1 Historic Overview of Equine Assisted Therapy.

This chapter is mainly taken from my final dissertation for my training as an Equine Assisted Therapist, (DAS). ***The specific uses and benefits of integrating Equine Assisted Therapy, linked with techniques of altered states of consciousness.**"*

Equine Assisted Therapy, (EAT), is exactly what is sounds to be, using horses to assist with therapy.

As with the history of trance states, this is also not new:

The therapeutic benefits of the horse were recognized starting from the year 460 BC.

Hippocrates spoke of the healthy pace of the horse.[46]

Ancient Greek literature mentioned the use of horse-back riding as therapy. In 600 BC, Orbasis documented the therapeutic benefit of horse riding.[47]

And later the Romans recognised the therapeutic value of horseback riding.[48]

The claimed benefits of therapeutic riding have been dated back to 17th century literature where it is documented that it was prescribed for gout, neurological disorder and low morale.[49]

---

[46] Asocequinoterapia 15 12 2016 The history and development of Equine Therapy
http://www.asocequinoterapia.org/english/Historia.htm Retrieved 15.05.2016

[47] Equestrian Therapy - 15.05.2016 History of equestrian therapy (Equestrian Therapy -
http://www.equestriantherapy.com/ Retrieved 15.05.2016

[48] R.D.A 16.05.2016
https://en.wikipedia.org/wiki/Riding_for_the_Disabled_Association Retrieved 16.05.2016

[49] Willis, D. A. (1997). Animal therapy. Rehabilitation Nursing, 22(2), 78-81, quoted in Wikipedia 'History'

Early studies to prove the therapeutic value of riding were started in 1875. The same year the French neurologist, Chassaignac, discovered that a horse in action improved the balance, motion and control muscle of his patients.

Their experiences convinced him that riding, improved mood, which was particularly beneficial for paraplegics and patients with other neurological disorders.[50]

More recently, in the United Kingdom, Miss Olive Sands MCSP took her horses to the Oxford Hospital to provide riding for the rehabilitation of Soldiers wounded in the trenches during the First World War.[51]

In Scandinavia, during the outbreak of poliomyelitis in 1946, equestrian therapy was introduced.[52]

---

https://en.wikipedia.org/wiki/Equine-assisted_therapy
Retrieved 16.05.2016
[50] See 45
[51] See 47
[52] See 46

The founding of the Community Association of Riding of the Disabled (CARD) started therapeutic riding in the USA and Canada in 1960. It has become a recreation and a motivational activity for the disabled while at the same time a therapy for them.[53]

Classic Equine Therapy in Europe has reflected the widespread German model since 1960, whose fundamental principles are the relationship between the movements of the horse and the patient's response to the treatment.[54]

Hippotherapy as currently practiced was developed in the 1960s, when it began to be used in Germany, Austria, and Switzerland as an adjunct to traditional physical therapy.[55]

---

[53] See 46
[54] See 45
[55] AHA "The History of Hippotherapy". American Hippotherapy Association http://www.americanhippotherapyassociation.org/ quoted in Wikipedia 'History' https://en.wikipedia.org/wiki/Equine-assisted_therapy Retrieved 16.05.2016

The oldest-known center for disabled people in the US was established in 1969 Michigan, the Cheff Therapeutic Riding center for the Handicapped.[56]

From there, a long time expert in the field of equine facilitated psychotherapy, and NARHA professional, Barbara Rector, introduced the healing benefits of horses to Sierra Tucson, an exclusive drug and alcohol addiction centre.[57]

She, (Barbara Rector) then went on to found, Therapeutic Riding of Tucson, Inc. (TROT) which she co-founded in 1974 with Nancy McGibbon and at Sierra Tucson Hospitals.

---

[56] See 46
[57] Claire Dorotik-Nana, LMFT 15.05.2016 PsychCentral, A Short History of Equine Therapy by By Claire Dorotik-Nana, LMFT http://blogs.psychcentral.com/equine-therapy/2011/01/a-short-history-of-equine-therapy/ 15.05.2016

Here she introduced and developed therapeutic work with horses and the practice of Equine Facilitated Psychotherapy.[58]

The first centre of its kind to partake in this ground breaking approach, Sierra Tucson soon also became recognized as a pioneer in the world of addiction recovery.[59]

10.2 Equine Assisted Therapy and Psychotherapy.

As is noted above, the uses of horses as partners for helping those with psychological problems has been seen to have existed for quite some time.

---

[58] Hacienda River 15 05 2016 - The Hacienda at the River http://haciendariver.watermarkcommunities.com/barbara-rector/ Retrieved 15 05 2016

[59] See 56

Within the framework of our therapy centre, my wife, our horse trainer and myself have been running psychotherapy groups using horses for nearly eight years.

What inspired my wife to create these groups was her personal experience of the sensitivity of the horse to read her mood and reactions better than she was able to.

Horses are, by their nature, being prey, hypersensitive to everything in their environments. However, they are big, heavy, strong, protective of their own space, have big strong teeth and can kill a human with a well-aimed kick.

On the other hand, being herd animals, (generally); sociable, communicative, intelligent, kind, willing, hierarchical, (trained to follow the orders of their leaders) and, for the most part, good natured.

It is this combination of inherent attributes that lends them so well to the therapeutic work.

135

To be able to; approach, contact, hold, attach, lead, stroke, brush and direct this massive, powerful beast, has multiple and various benefits.

However, for integrating in a hypnotherapeutic process, these attributes are used in a totally different fashion ...

10.3 Hypnotherapeutic Benefits of working with Horses.

As already mentioned above, techniques of altered states of consciousness are useful because they bypass the conscious levels of defence of the patient.

We can hence, plant certain suggestions, that although the conscious mind might be aware of, it is directly to the unconscious part of the patient that we are addressing.

Certain aspects of Equine Assisted Therapy, can certainly help in the availability of the patient towards the therapy on course:

For instance, that the patient can feel that being on a horse gives them a feeling of power, confidence, autonomy,

And that being outside of a formal psychotherapeutic space can relax the patient, and hence leave them much more open to psychotherapeutic interventions, etc.

These above benefits apply generally to working with horses.

However, it is the possibility to use the symbolic force of the horse, within the hypnotic induction that lends itself so powerfully to the technique.

First, I have found, that by placing the patient on horseback, and having the horse move, while using normal hypnotic verbal techniques, most patients, quickly fall into a trance state.

Not only that, the bilateral alternate stimulation, of the walking horse, totally mimics the techniques used to activate the deep change process that is at the root of the EMDR and ABS therapeutic procedures.

Hence, even if one chooses to pass on all other parts of this therapeutic technique, we can still benefit from one of its fundamental concepts – that alternative, bilateral stimulation helps relax the patient and supports the deep process of change.

Yet, this is just the first of many benefits of this shared technique.

10.4 Merging with the Horse

As the experience of being on a horse walking, also mimics the person's own experience of walking, with the suggestion that the rider and the horse can start to merge, to become part of the same whole, it is relatively easy, for the rider to feel the separation between him and the horse to become less and less clear, and to finally, feel as if the two are, in fact joining.

As we have noted above, we invest many positive traits onto the image of a horse.

It then becomes more or less obvious, depending on the particular problem of the patient, to find a specific trait, that exists in their image of the horse, that they can, due to the fact that they are now intimately linked to the horse, be capable to integrate that trait into themselves.

One must realise the potency of this psychological manoeuvre. We all have defence mechanisms that protect us from accepting things within ourselves that do not fit with our own self-images.

We are suggesting to the patient that they have attributes which they clearly feel that they neither have, nor could possibly, ever have.

Hence, in normal situations, even in a 'normal or usual' hypnotic setting, to suggest that, within themselves, they have these possibilities, would, more than likely, awaken a strong defence mechanism, to block this going too far into their psyche.

By using their connection to the horse, an animal that is known to have these possibilities, we bypass this defence mechanism.

They cannot deny that the horse is like that, and because they are now, to some degree, fused, even integrated into it, if the horse is like that, they too can be the same.

So, every positive aspect of the horse, that it is; strong, intelligent, brave, confident, social, caring, supportive, attentive, adaptable, able to run or to fight, able to fight for its place, yet able to accept its position and the control and judgement of a hierarchical superior, etc., can be offered to the patient as his own.

11 Hypnosis and Virtual Reality – The Future

One might well argue that hypnosis is, in itself a form of virtual reality. Patients during a hypnotical trance can fully experience all forms of sensory perceptions; sight, sound, smell, touch, taste and movement.

However, there are some members of the population, for a variety of reasons are not capable to generate these experiences, even under the competent hand of an experienced hypnotherapist.

Also, many others, do not, nor might not have access to a hypnotherapist. And, although there exists many and varied hypnotic recordings, it can be particularly difficult for the person to create the necessary environment, externally and internally, which is necessary to achieve a satisfactory result.

12 A hypothesis on how and why EMDR works

EMDR and possibly other forms of trauma therapy which use the ABS, (Alternative Bilateral Stimulation), have a proven rate of success.

However, this success has not, to my knowledge benefitted from a coherent reflection of what is happening and how it might work.

My reflection is based on the understanding that the left and right hemispheres of the brain, serve different functions; the right side more emotional, while the left side is more for analytic processing.

I would suggest that strong experiences first and mainly activate the right hemisphere, which is then passed on to the left hemisphere for processing.

From there onwards the experience is treated between the two hemispheres, in a form of ping-pong between two types of processing.

Reexperiencing, then reflection, reexperiencing, reflection, and so on, and so forth.

Until all the elements are 'ground down' and capable of being 'digested' and integrated into the system or let go and forgotten.

In a moment of extreme emotion, trauma, as the experience is too important to deal with in the moment, one experiences sensory overload, and the system shuts down.

However, the person, in the course of being traumatised, is still aware of what is happening around them. In fact, they are, if anything, hyper-aware; every sound, smell, image and sensation is faithfully recorded.

On the other hand, their normal thinking, processing functions are totally disrupted.

The experience is too extreme to handle, too extreme to be understood, too extreme to deal with.

What one can ascertain from this is that the right hemisphere is over-operating, experiencing and recording all the events in the smallest detail.

While the left hemisphere is to some large degree blocked from its usual level of functioning.

Researching this hypothesis, I came across the wide-ranging paper of
Heath A. Demaree and his colleagues on Brain Lateralization of Emotional Processing,[60]

---

[60] Demaree, H. A. et al, Brain Lateralization of Emotional Processing: Historical Roots and a Future Incorporating "Dominance"
https://pdfs.semanticscholar.org/0f66/c2791e5d549aed4b6316 7a59b69a326bcd30.pdf retrieved 12.07.2019

"Observations of a direct link between emotion processing and the right hemisphere were made nearly 100 years ago.

The valence hypothesis postulates that the right hemisphere is specialized for negative emotion."

Also, a most interesting research into "Neurobiological Correlates of EMDR Monitoring" which came to these conclusions:

"Our findings point to a highly significant activation shift following EMDR therapy from limbic regions with high emotional valence to cortical regions with higher cognitive and associative valence."[61]

---

[61] PLoS One. 2012; 7(9): e45753. Published online 2012 Sep 26. doi: 10.1371/journal.pone.0045753 PMCID: PMC3458957 PMID: 23049852 Neurobiological Correlates of EMDR Monitoring – An EEG Study
https://www.ncbi.nlm.nih.gov/pmc/articles/PMC3458957/
retrieved 27.07.2019

With all this in mind, if we can accept the concept that trauma can overstimulate the right side of the brain and hinder the functioning of the left, where does this lead us?

First of all it can open up a very simple understanding of why the symptoms of PTSD exist and what are their function? (Yes, I did say that these symptoms have a function).

I general, the symptoms of PTSD all, on some level are a reactivation of the traumatic event; flashbacks, nightmares, hypersensitivity to sounds and movements etc.

The right hemisphere re-serves the event to the left side, to start the ping-pong process of grinding up, (or down) the traumatic events, but the 'ball' is too big and too heavy, and the left side chooses not to 'play'.

This is where therapy comes in.

147

By helping the patient to consciously reactivate the traumatic experience, (right hemisphere) and to talk about the surrounding events, before and after and their thoughts etc., (left hemisphere), the therapist forces the both sides to interact and the process of dealing with and integrating the experience to advance.

However, the intellectual defences of the left hemisphere or the re-traumatisation and subsequent emotional overloading of the right, are natural obstacles to the therapeutic process.

Hypnotic techniques can be interesting as they can reactivate the memories in a more controlled fashion and even work towards changing the fixed memory experience.

As the experience changes, the intense emotional charge linked to the original events becomes more mobile and left side can begin to undertake its function of processing and integration.

What is even more interesting when using ABS is that, even before invoking the traumatic events, (directly or, as I choose often to work, indirectly), both hemispheres are equally activated.

This external, forced activation, means that as soon as the trauma is evoked, the left hemisphere as already active and functioning to deal with the material.

Hence, the 'usual' and natural reticence to intellectually open oneself to the extent of these events is bypassed and these therapeutic approaches prove themselves as particularly efficient in dealing with trauma.

13 The Pinch

I have added these extra lines about 'The Pinch', so as to further clarify the range of uses of this induction.

I have written above, one can use this technique to relax and calm oneself in many stressful situations; speaking before an audience, during exams, before and during an interview, etc., etc.

To illustrate this, I will offer a personal anecdote.

My wife and I were working together for the Dr. G. Salem, who had taken me on as a trainee and had then convinced my wife to join him in his small group clinic.

We were returning from lunch, chatting. When I felt something tickling my hand, so I shook my hand a little violently to remove what-ever it was.

Bad idea.

I had upset a wasp, and being upset, it did what any self-respecting wasp would do – it stung me.

And as anyone that has had their finger stung by a wasp will know, it rather hurt.

So, as I was walking and talking to my wife, trying to cope with the pain, I reflected that I had been leading an auto-hypnosis group for over a year, and maybe it might be a good moment to try and put that discipline into practice.

And so, I pressed my two index and thumbs together, concentrated on the contact and focused the rest of my attention on the sensations coming from my pricked finger.

The pain quickly transformed into a combination of heat and an amusing sensation of vibration.

Not to forget, during the same time I was walking down quite a steep hill, listening and responding to our conversation.

151

Just before arriving at work, my wife was a little surprised that I wasn't thinking to go straight into the next-door chemist shop.

"What for?" I asked.

"Something for the pain."

"But there is no more pain."

"Well, at least for some disinfectant."

As with most husbands, I found it easier to agree to her concerns and have my injury correctly treated.

The pain never returned, and the sting healed at an amazing rate.

Update.
Last week, (17th of July 2019), I was swimming in the ocean near St. Tropez, when, for my sins, I was stung by a jellyfish. – And it hurt!

However, being totally into finishing this book, I didn't hesitate before re-introducing myself to the Pinch.

By the time that I reached the shore, a matter of several minutes, some blustering had begun to appear and my wife was rushing up to me to inspect the damage.

"How much does it hurt?" She inquired.

"Not so much", I responded.

"Doesn't it sting?"

"Actually, no", I might have been as surprised as she was.

For the next few hours the skin was a little tender, so I was careful not to rub anything against it, but the pain had totally ceased.

By the evening, it was all but healed.

A miracle? – No, I don't think so.

Could there be a scientific explanation how my sting had healed in just a few hours?

I do think so.

When we have damage to the skin, we release histamine.

The American Academy of Allergy, Asthma & Immunology explain it this way.[62]

"What Makes Us Itch?

Itching can be caused by many different things including allergies, insect bites, dry skin or illness.

Itch and pain are closely linked in the brain.

The reflex to pain is to withdraw.
The reflex to itch is to scratch. This reflex is a protective response developed to help animals remove parasites from their skin.

---

[62]What makes us itch? https://www.aaaai.org/conditions-and-treatments/library/allergy-library/what-makes-us-itch retrieved 29.07.2019

That's why even a slight movement of hairs is enough to make you want to scratch.

Itching is often triggered by histamine, a chemical in the body associated with immune responses.

It causes the itch and redness you see with insect bites, rashes and skin dryness or damage.

Histamine is released by the body during allergic reactions, such as those to pollen, food, latex and medications."
    – And wasp and jellyfish stings.

My hypothesis goes something like this:

By suppressing the pain reaction in the brain, the histamine trigger is also blocked.

It is the histamine that creates the secondary inflammation and the itching.

Without this, as long as one does nothing to reactivate this mechanism, the poison,

(wasp or jellyfish sting), is quite quickly absorbed into the body, and almost immediately there are neither pain nor soreness.

14 The Flower

This section is taken from chapter 14 of my book on hypnosis, 'Remember'[63]

14: The Flower

[Each chapter begins and ends with several anecdotes, two, loosely taken from my therapeutic practice, and one from my own personal life. I have removed the professional stories but have kept that of my own].

My wife is twenty-eight weeks pregnant with our first child. She is confined to bed-rest, due to crises of contractions. She is often in great pain, but, worse than that, she is scared for the health and safety of our baby.

---

[63] Gary Edward Gedall. *Remember.* From Words to Worlds, Lausanne 2003 – 11

Yet another series of contractions start. She tenses up, the pain and fear mount.

I run a warm bath; she tries to relax a little…

****

Pain and tension, whether physical, emotional or psychological, form a perfect, vicious circle. Whichever comes first, if it succeeds to activate the second, unless and until this mutually re-enforcing system is interrupted, pain and tension will continue to worsen.

However, to try and block, or force to re-open, or to relax, will only activate the same mechanism which will resist and thence re-enforce the tension and pain.

Patience and gentle coaxing are needed to calm the little, scared animal in self-inflicted pain into trusting enough to release its grip and to let itself fall into the protective, comforting arms that await it.

158

"For this exercise allow your hand(s) to close into a quite tight fist. If you also have a pain that might be linked to tension, allow your mind to also notice this. This applies equally to emotional or intellectual tensions.

During this induction your hand can open more and more, following the course of the opening of the flower. You might very likely feel a releasing of the other tensions during and after this induction."

The Flower

The night is cold and dark;
The moon is high;
The stars dance.
All is calm,
Serene,
Asleep.
The flower sleeps,
Its head bent low,
Its petals tightly folded.

The dark becomes less clear,
The cold more intense.
The moon descends
And stars begin to fade.
The world holds its breath.
Tension.
The flower shivers
With fear,
The head even lower,
Petals even more closed

The sky whispers of light;
The moon falls;
The stars become vague memories.

160

The cold bites;
The day waits to enter.
The tension increases.
The flower shivers
With anticipation.
It rests totally immobile;
Head and petals.

Bands of radiance cross the horizon;
The sun promises.
Clouds exist.
The day begins,
The cold blunts,
The tension relaxes,
The flower shivers
Into awakening;
The head senses the dream of change,
The petals stiffen

The blue pales,
Washed by the light of sun.
The day has awakened.
The air excites,
The cold fades,
The flower responds;

161

Its body enters into movement,
Lifting the head,
The petals sense the change.

The sun floats gently into day,
Cushioned by a quiet haze.
The air exults the birth.
The temperature is warming.
The flower responds;
The stem directs the
Raising head in the direction
Of the light;
First response.

The sun passes the horizon,
The day has begun,
The air loses its last chill,
The birds break into gentle song;
The head straightens,
The very tips of the petals
Unclench.

The sun mounts,
The insects stir,
A quiet blue invades the sky.

162

The stem is sure;
The first layer of petals
Begin to separate from the head –
Gently, little by little,
The silken arms
Extend.

The day has fully arrived;
The sun has settled
On its skyward course
A warm breeze
Floats
Gently
Across.
The flower
Breathes
The first prayer.

Little by little,
Inch by inch,
The petals
Release their tension,
Relaxing,
One after another
Opening,

Softening;
The next layer,
Already prepared,
Actively,
Impatiently,
Awaiting each its turn.
Ready,
Release,
Relax…
And again,
      And again,
            And again.
Ready,
      Ready,
            Ready.
Release,
      Release,
            Release.
Relax,
      Relax,
            Relax.

The day advances;
Birds fly;
The sun imposes his
Presence.

164

The flower
Dances,
Loosening her veils;
The last layers of petals
Open,
Revealing
Inner secrets

The day hangs heavily;
The sun is in his power.
He reigns down
His golden manna.
The flower responds,
Absorbing,
Enriching,
Opening her deepest,
Richest self.
And so –
There she is;
Open,
Vulnerable,
Pure,
Relaxed.

For so is the state
In which
She can profit
The most
From all
That life
Has to offer.

****

My wife arrives at term.

We continue using hypnosis at the clinic.
The midwives question whether she is really
in labour, as she shows no signs of pain or
discomfort.

Our daughter is now twenty years old – [as
of 08.2019].

Discussion:

Tension begets pain and fear and sickness
and suffering.
It also closes us from our free-flowing
energies.
Relax and release these tensions;
Trust life that if you open to it,
It will feed and nourish you.
Set free the suffering,
Liberate pleasure,
Inhale life;
Exist –
Full.

Other Works

REMEMBER

Stories and poems for self-help and self-development based on techniques of Ericksonian and auto-hypnosis

Dusk falls, the world shrinks little by little into a smaller and smaller circle as the light continues to diminish.

The centre of this world is illuminated by a small, crackling sun; the flames dance, and the rough faces of the people gathered there are lit by the fire of their expectations.

The old man will begin to speak, he will explain to them how the world is, how it was, how it was created. He will help them understand how things have a sense, an order, a way that they need to be.

He will clarify the sources of un-wellness and unhappiness, what is sickness, where it comes from, how to notice it and… how to heal it.

To heal the sick, he will call forth the forces of the invisible realms, maybe he will sing, certainly he will talk, and talk, and talk.

Since the beginning of time we have gathered round those who can bring us the answers to our questions and the means to alleviate our sufferings.

This practice has not fundamentally changed since the earliest times; in every era, continent and culture we have found and continue to find these experiences.

In this, amongst the oldest of the healing traditions, he has succeeded to meld modern therapy theories and techniques with stories and poems of the highest quality.

With much humanity, clinical vignettes, common sense and lots of humour, the reader is gently carried from situation to situation.

Whether the problems described concern you directly, indirectly or not at all, you will surely find interest and benefits from the wealth of insights and advices contained within and the conscious or unconscious positive changes through reading the stories and poems.

The Zen Approach to Modern Living Vol 1

Fundamentals, Family & Friends

Life is often experienced as a series of conflicts and aggressions, both from the outside and within ourselves.

The Zen Approach to Modern Living series, will lead you towards a more harmonious way of dealing with the many, complex and competing elements of your daily life.

These conflicts leave us exhausted, depressed, angry, and feeling generally unhappy and unfulfilled.

Being more in harmony with yourself will bring more happiness, more energy and open up the route to self-fulfilment.

Volume 1 covers; an introduction to the basic concepts, our relationship with ourselves, our family, (partner, children, parents, brothers, sisters and in-laws), friends and enemies.

Plus, plus, plus, A Bonus Chapter: My Deepest, Darkest, Secret.

171

The Zen Approach to Modern Living Vol 2

Work - Paradise or Purgatory?

This second volume in the Zen Approach series continues in the same style as volume one…

We spend most of our adult life at work.

We will all havc colleagues, bosses, and often subordinates

Hopefully, these people will be polite and professional.

Some of them won't.

This book will help you:
-Choose the best type of job for you.
-How to approach a new job
&
-How to deal with difficult colleagues, bosses, & subordinates

Rich with practical advice, images and interesting and amusing stories, the Zen Approach Vol 2, will help yet entertain you towards your Paradise of a workplace.

172

The Zen Approach to Low Impact Training and Sports

A simple method for achieving a healthy body and a healthy mind

Many of us approach our fitness and sports activities in an aggressive and competitive fashion.

And even if we feel that we succeed to break out of our comfort zones and win against ourselves or our opponent, there is an important cost to bear.

This level of violence that we have come to accept, so as to reach our goals is also an aggression against ourselves.

By removing this need to 'win at any price', and tuning in with our bodies and emotions, we can achieve an enormous amount, all the while being in harmony with our mind, body and spirit.

The Zen approach to Low Impact Training and Sports, is a new softer approach where you can have the best of all worlds.

Island of Serenity Book 1
The Island of Survival

Suicide

Pierre-Alain James 'Faron' Ferguson is about to commit suicide, in his suicide note he attempts to understand how he has come to have wrecked not only his own life, but also all of those around him.

Pierre-Alain James 'Faron' Ferguson finds himself in a type of 'no-mans-land', between here and there, he must accept to visit 7 islands before he will be allowed to continue on to his next steps.

The islands are named; Survival, Pleasure, Esteem, Love, Expression, Insight and lastly, the Island of Serenity

The Early Years:

Pierre-Alain James 'Faron' Ferguson is born into a well-to-do household of a factory owner, Scottish father and mother of a noble French family

He, and his younger brother Jay, grow up in a home of two distant but invested parents. Already, the first, small stones of his future problems are being put into place.

The Island of Survival:

Faron finds himself on the first of the seven islands, transformed into a prehistoric human form, he must learn how to interact with the local environment and the early humanoid tribe.

Here, he must reconnect with his instinct of survival.

175

Island of Serenity Book 2
Sun & Rain

This is the second chapter of Faron's life history.

After his parents learn of his relationship with Angelique, they have two interesting reactions:

First they send the two boys off to America for the summer holidays to live and work on a western ranch

Then they enrol them in a Scottish boarding school to begin at the beginning of the next school term.

St. Joseph's wasn't such a bad experience, especially after Faron starts a friendship with the two boys that are to become his best friends.

Duncan, a kind and gentle Christian and Mike, an intelligent, hard worker from a quite poor environment.

However, it is his growing interest for Angelique that haunts his psyche.

An attachment supported by his old nurse Marie-Madeleine, and with a certain indifference by his father.

His mother's reaction is something else again, and any means to keep them apart and put a stop to this relationship are fair game, even if it means sending him to her unacceptable sister or a skiing holiday in Switzerland.

But, as they say, love will find a way

Island of Serenity Book 3
The Island of Pleasure
Vol 1 Venice

Part 1.

Faron finds himself in a past version of
Venice, as the owner of an old but grand
hotel that doubles as the meeting place for
the wealthy men of the City and the high-
class escort girls that live in the
establishment.

Faron can do anything that he likes without
limitation or cost. Not only can he avail
himself of the girls, but can eat and drink,
without limit, but never suffer from a
hangover, nor gain a gram.

So why has the enigmatic guide brought
him here, and will his limitless access to
life's offerings really bring him the pleasure
that he is destined to experience?

Part 2.

Faron is transformed into an adolescent tom boy. In this more modern version of Venice, 'he' has just 7 days to be made into a high-class escort girl.

What does this experience and the intrigues of the other persons within his sphere, mean for him, on his continuing quest to understand, and to experience, Pleasure?

Island of Serenity Book 4
The Island of Pleasure
Vol 2 Japan

Faron finds himself in the mystery of a long-ago Japan, in the body of a young, trainee Geisha.

Who is this sad, young man that he must help to find back his pleasure in life?

Why must he hide the identity of his mother, from the rest of the world?

Why was the love of his mother's life, stolen away by her sister, known to all as Madame Butterfly?

What part does the feudal lord of the region have in all this?

And how does Faron finally succeed to find the key to rediscovering pleasure in his life?

Island of Serenity Book 5
Rise and Fall

In this the 5th book of the series, we watch as Faron grows from an adolescent into a young, driven man.

He begins by escaping to New York, before starting his University career, finding back his two school, best friends, Duncan and Mike.

After graduating, the three find themselves setting up a business, manufacturing, buying and importing goods from Indonesia.

Success seems to be just around the corner, but Faron cannot help himself. Bitterness and betrayal, hound him like a hungry dog.

To destroy, his own best friend, is not an act to take lightly, but take it, he does.

And what of Angelique, and his daughter Aideen? He is still emotionally entangled, but is that a good thing, or a very bad thing?

Only time will tell.

181

Island of Serenity Book 6
The Island of Esteem pt1

The Knight's Tale

Faron, our anti-hero, finds himself transported into the body of Sir Lancelot, at the court of King Arthur.

He is on the quest to heal his self-esteem, but the knight, although noble and brave, is also a flawed human-being.

One person that avoids emotional conflicts but cannot escape his passion for Guinevere.

The knight has lost his memory, so he cannot remember how or why he has come to this point in his history.

And who is Al, his faithful squire who has helped him steal a magical sceptre from his supposed best friend, King Galahaut?

Follow Lancelot through his tortured romantic journey, in a world of court intrigue, magic and heroism.

Island of Serenity Book 7
The Island of Esteem pt2

Le Morte D'Arthur

In this second and concluding volume of the Island of Esteem, we follow Al, as he continues to demonstrate to Faron, just what it means to be a hero.

Lancelot still is troubled by his past and present inability to impose himself, in any situation other than battle.

We get to understand how it was that Lancelot was forgiven by Guinevere, and why Arthur accepted to call on his help to retrieve the Uffington sceptre.

And how and why Al, chose and succeeded to steal it.

Also, how and why, he will be motivated to steal it, not just and second, but also a third time.

183

We follow the magical manipulations of Merlin and Morgan le Fey.

And finally, what happens to Lancelot and Al, before, during and after the final battle between Arthur and Mordred.

Emotional Rescue

For almost 50 years I have been writing
about Longing, Love and Loss.

Pleasure and Purgatory.

Tears of sadness, joy or laughter.

Here, I would like to share with you a
lifetime of my connection with the
emotional treasure house of relationships.

Through poetry, prose, stories and songs, I
will offer to lead you on a journey to the
deepest parts of my own soul.

Adventures with the Master

Dhargey was a sickly child, or so his parents treated him.

He was too weak to join the army or work in the fields or even join the monastery as a normal trainee monk.

To explain to the 'Young Master' why he should be accepted into the order with a lightened program, he was forced to accompany the revered old man a little ways up the mountain.

As his parents watched him leave; somewhere they felt that they would never see their sickly, fragile boy ever again, somewhere they were totally right.

He was a happy, healthy seven year old until he witnessed the riders, dressed in red and black, destroying his village and murdering his parents; the trauma cut deep into his psyche.

186

Only the chance meeting with a wandering monk could set him back onto the road towards health and serenity.

Through meditation, initiations, stories, taming wild horses, becoming a monkey, mastering the staff and the sword; the future 'Young Master' prepares to face his greatest demon.

Two men, two journeys; one goal…

Picturing the Mind

Vol 1

A simple model capable to explain the functioning and dysfunctioning of the human psyche.

Introduction to the Field theory of Human Functioning

For the average man and woman in the street, the complex and competing theories and models of the human psyche; its development, functioning and dis-functioning are often unhelpful for their understanding of themselves.

This becomes even more problematic when they find themselves in difficulty, as often, even the mental health professionals, who are experts in their own fields, find themselves at a loss to communicate successfully how and why the patent is unwell and what needs to happen to find or regain a healthy balance.

188

This opens up the question; 'is it possible to image a simple, single model, accessible to everyone, to explain the development, functioning and dis-functioning of the human psyche?'

One that builds on existing theories and models, benefitting from the mass of experience and research of 'modern western' psychological concepts and ideas, but also integrating traditional visions of the human psyche and modern theories from the physical sciences.

Picturing the Mind, is an attempt to answer to this need.

189

Picturing the Mind
Vol 2

The second volume following on from the
initial concepts will reflect on such subjects
as:

> Relationships
> Exchanging energy
> Heart & Soul
> Recuperation
> Subjective constructions
> An unconscious yes, an unconscious

no

> Me, myself and everyone else
> Circles in circles, the micro level
> Circles in circles, the macro level
> Intuition
> Metaphysical reflections

Picturing the Mind

Vol 3

Will deal with:

Psychopathology

Traditional psychotherapy
&
Alternative therapeutic approaches.

www.ingramcontent.com/pod-product-compliance
Lightning Source LLC
Chambersburg PA
CBHW061744120626
46550CB00005B/1887